The Teaching from Grigori Grabovoi
"Deliverance and Harmonious Development"

Grigori Grabovoi

Restoration of the Human Organism through Concentration on Numbers

The restorative number sequences in this book
were given by Grigori Grabovoi in 1999.

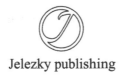

Jelezky publishing

Restoration of the Human Organism through
Concentration on Numbers

Edition: 2011-1, 29.08.2011

TABLE OF CONTENTS

Page(Row)

Introduction..**27**

Chapter 1   CRITICAL CONDITIONS – 1258912 .....**36(07)**
Cardiac arrest – 8915678 ....36(10)
Cardiovascular insufficiency,
acute (Heart failure, acute) – 1895678...............................36(17)
Respiratory failure, acute – 1257814 ....36(25)
Traumatic shock, shock and shock–like
conditions – 1895132...37(02)

Chapter 2   TUMORS – 8214351 ....**38(07)**
Cancer, bladder – 89123459 ....38(10)
Cancer, bone – 1234589..38(14)
Cancer, breast – 5432189..38(20)
Cancer, colon (Colorectal cancer) – 5821435......................38(26)
Cancer, esophageal – 8912567...38(33)
Cancer, extrahepatic bile duct – 5789154............................39(01)
Cancer, gallbladder – 8912453 ....39(06)
Cancer, kidney – 56789108 ....39(12)
Cancer, lips – 1567812..39(16)
Cancer, liver – 5891248 ....39(19)
Cancer, lung (Pulmonary cancer) – 4541589 – See Chpt 7:
Respiratory Diseases, Lung cancer......................................39(24)
Cancer, major duodenal papilla – 8912345 ....39(27)
Cancer, mouth and throat – 1235689 ....39(32)
Cancer, ovarian – 4851923 ....40(01)
Cancer, pancreatic – 8125891...40(05)
Cancer, penis – 8514921..40(10)
Cancer, prostate – 4321890...40(13)
Cancer, salivary gland – 9854321...40(17)
Cancer, skin – 8148957..40(21)
Cancer, small intestines – 5485143.......................................40(28)
Cancer, stomach – 8912534 ....40(32)

Cancer, testicular – 5814321.. 41(03)
Cancer, thyroid – 5814542... 41(08)
Cancer, ureter – 5891856 .... 41(12)
Cancer, vaginal and of the external genitals – 2589121 .... 41(16)
Cancer, vulva – 5148945 .... 41(20)
Hematosarcoma and Lymphoma – 54321451 –
See Chpt 10: Blood Diseases: Hemoblastosis outside of
bone marrow, Hematosarcoma, and Lymphoma
(Lymphocytoma)... 41(23)
Leukemia – 5481347– see Chpt 10:
Blood Diseases, Leukemia... 41(27)
Lymphogranulomatosis (Hodgkin's disease)
– 4845714– see Chpt 10: Blood Diseases,
Lymphogranulomatosis.. 41(30)
Lymphoma of the skin – 5891243 .... 41(34)
Melanoma – 5674321 .... 42(03)
Mesothelioma – 58912434.. 42(08)
Neuroblastoma – 8914567.. 42(11)
Plasmocytoma, Multiple Myeloma,
Non-Hodgkin Lymphoma – 8432184 – See Chpt 10:
Blood Diseases, Paraproteinemia producing tumors .... 42(16)
Rhabdomyosarcoma in children – 5671254 .... 42(20)
Sarcoma, Kaposi's – 8214382... 42(26)
Sarcoma, soft-tissue – 54321891 .... 42(31)
Tumor, adrenal – 5678123 .... 43(01)
Tumor, brain – 5451214– See Chpt 18:
Neurological Diseases, Brain tumor .... 43(06)
Tumor, brain or spinal cord – 5431547.................................... 43(09)
Tumor, islet cell – 8951432 .... 43(13)
Tumor, nasal cavity and paranasal sinuses – 8514256 .... 43(18)
Tumor, nasopharynx – 5678910 .... 43(22)
Tumor, parathyroid – 1548910 .... 43(26)
Tumor, peripheral nervous system –
514832182 – See Chpt 18: Neurological Diseases,
Tumor, peripheral nervous system.. 43(31)
Tumor, spinal cord – 51843210 – See Chpt 18: Neurological
Diseases, Tumor, spinal cord .... 44(01)
Tumor, uterus – 9817453 .... 44(04)

© Г. П. Грабовой, 1999

Chapter 3   SEPSIS – 58143212.................................**45(07)**
Sepsis (Blood poisoning)
– acute – 8914321; chronic – 8145421 .... 45(10)

Chapter 4   DIC-SYNDROME – 5148142...................**46(07)**
Disseminated Intravascular Coagulation
(DIC syndrome) – 8123454 .... 46(11)

**Chapter 5   DISEASES OF THE
                 CARDIOVASCULAR
                 SYSTEM – 1289435**...................................**47(07)**
Aneurysm, aortic – 48543218 – see Chpt 22:
Surgeries, Aneurysm... 47(11)
Aneurysm, cardiac – 9187549 – see Chpt 22: Surgeries .... 47(14)
Arrhythmia (Cardiac dysrhythmia) – 8543210...................... 47(17)
Atherosclerosis – 54321898... 47(22)
Autonomic neuropathy (Vegetovascular dystonia)
– 8432910.. 47(29)
Cardiac asthma – 8543214... 48(01)
Cardialgia – 8124567... 48(06)
Cardiomyopathy (Myocardiopathy) – 8421432.................... 48(11)
Cardiosclerosis – 4891067... 48(18)
Circulatory failure – 85432102.. 48(23)
Collapse – 8914320.. 48(29)
Congenital heart defect – 9995437 .... 48(34)
Cor pulmonale (Pulmonary heart disease) – 5432111 .... 49(05)
Endocarditis – 8145999 .... 49(11)
Heart blocks – 9874321 .... 49(16)
Heart defect, acquired – 8124569 .... 49(19)
Heart failure (Cardiac failure) – 8542196............................. 49(23)
Hypertension (High blood pressure) – 8145432.................... 49(27)
Hypertensive crisis – 5679102... 49(30)
Hypotension (Low blood pressure) – 8143546...................... 50(01)
Ischemic heart disease – IHD
(Coronary heart disease) – 1454210 .... 50(05)
Myocardial infarction (Heart attack) – 8914325 .... 50(11)
Myocardiodystrophy – 8432110.. 50(17)
Myocarditis – 85432104 .... 50(21)
Neurocirculatory dystonia – 5432150................................... 50(24)

Occlusion of major arteries – 81543213 – see Chpt 22:
Surgeries, Occlusion of major arteries .... 50(31)
Pericarditis – 9996127 .... 50(34)
Pulmonary edema (Lung edema) – 54321112 .... 51(01)
Rheumatic heart disease (Rheumatic fever)– 5481543 –
see Chpt 6: Rheumatic Diseases: Rheumatic fever .... 51(06)
Stenocardia (Angina pectoris) – 8145999 .... 51(10)
Systemic vasculitis – 1894238 – see Chpt 6:
Rheumatic Diseases, Systemic vasculitis .... 51(15)
Thrombophlebitis – 1454580 – see Chpt 22:
Surgeries: Phlebothrombosis .... 51(18)
Varicosis – 4831388 – see Chpt 22: Surgeries, Varicosis .... 51(21)
Vascular crisis – 8543218 .... 51(24)
Vascular insufficiency – 8668888 .... 51(30)

Chapter 6   RHEUMATIC DISEASES – 8148888, JOINT DISEASES – 5421891

Chapter 6   **RHEUMATIC DISEASES – 8148888,**
      JOINT DISEASES – 5421891 .... 52(10)
Arthritis psoriatica – 0145421 .... 52(13)
Arthritis, degenerative (Osteoarthritis, Osteoarthrosis,
Arthrosis deformans, Degenerative joint disease) –
8145812 .... 52(17)
Arthritis, reactive – (Reiter's syndrome) – 4848111 .... 52(23)
Arthritis, rheumatoid – 8914201 .... 52(28)
Connective tissue disease, mixed
(Sharp's syndrome) – 1484019 .... 52(33)
Connective tissue diseases, diffuse – 5485812 .... 53(03)
Crystal Deposition Disease Syndrome – 0014235 .... 53(08)
Dermatomyositis (Polymyositis) – 5481234 .... 53(12)
Giant-cell Arteritis (Cranial arteritis, Temporal arteritis,
Horton's disease) – 9998102 .... 53(16)
Goodpasture's syndrome – 8491454 .... 53(22)
Hemorrhagic vasculitis
(Purpura Henoch-Schoenlein) – 8491234 .... 53(28)
Arthritis, infectious – 8111110 .... 53(33)
Lupus erythematosus – 8543148 .... 54(01)
Periarthritis – 4548145 .... 54(05)
Podagra (Gout) – 8543215 .... 54(09)
Polyarteritis nodosa (Periarteritis nodosa,
Kussmaul disease) – 54321894 .... 54(13)

Rheumatic heart disease (Rheumatic fever) – 5481543 .... 54(18)
Rheumatism, soft tissue near joint – 1489123 .... 54(33)
Sjoegren's syndrome
(Sicca syndrome, Mikulicz disease) – 4891456 .... 54(30)
Skleroderma, systemic – 1110006 .... 55(01)
Spondylitis ankylopoetica (Bechterew's disease,
Marie-Struempell disease) – 4891201 .... 55(06)
Systemic vasculitis (SV) – 1894238 .... 55(11)
Takayasu's arteritis – 8945432 .... 55(16)
Tendovaginitis – 1489154 .... 55(21)
Thrombangiitis obliterans (Buerger's disease) – 8945482 ..... 55(24)
Wegener's Granulomatosis – 8943568 .... 55(29)

Chapter 7   RESPIRATORY
DISEASES – 5823214 .... 56(07)

Anthracosis – 5843214 .... 56(10)
Asbestosis – 4814321 .... 56(14)
Aspergillosis – 481543271 .... 56(17)
Asthma, bronchial – 8943548 .... 56(22)
Bronchiolitis (Bronchioles, acute inflammation of) –
89143215 .... 56(26)
Bronchitis, acute – 4812567 .... 56(31)
Bronchitis, chronic – 4218910 .... 56(34)
Coal worker's pneumoconiosis
(Carboconiosis, Black lung disease) – 8148545 .... 57(03)
Emphysema, lung – 54321892 .... 57(08)
Lung fibrosis (Pneumosclerosis) – 9871234 .... 57(13)
Metalloconiosis – 4845584 .... 57(18)
Pleuritis (Pleurisy) – 4854444 .... 57(24)
Pneumoconiosis – 8423457 .... 57(28)
Pneumoconiosis of organic dust – 4548912 .... 57(33)
Pneumonia – 4814489 .... 58(01)
Pneumonitis, acute interstitial
(Hamman–Rich syndrome) – 4814578 .... 58(07)
Pulmonary cancer (lung cancer) – 4541589 .... 58(12)
Pulmonary candidiasis (Candidiasis of the lung) –
4891444 – See also Chpt 8: Digestive System, Candidiasis... 58(16)
Pulmonary infarction (Lung infarction) – 89143211 .... 58(21)
Sarcoidosis – 4589123 .... 58(25)

Silicatosis – 2224698 .... 58(31)
Silicosis (Potter's rot) – 4818912 .... 58(34)
Talcosis – 4845145 .... 59(04)
Tuberculosis, pulmonary – 8941234 .... 59(07)

**Chapter 8   DISEASES OF THE DIGESTIVE
                       SYSTEM – 5321482 .... 46**
Achalasia of cardia (Cardiospasm, Hiatal spasm,
Megaesophagus, Idiopathic dilation of esophagus) –
4895132 .... 60(07)
Achylia gastrica – 8432157 .... 60(10)
Amoebiasis – 1289145 – see Chpt 14: Infectious Diseases.... 60(24)
Amyloidosis – 5432185 .... 60(27)
Atonia of the esophagus and the stomach –
8123457 – see Dyskinesia of the digestive tract .... 60(31)
Beriberi – 3489112 .... 60(34)
Bronze diabetes – 5454589 .... 61(01)
Candidiasis (Thrush, Yeast infection) – 54842148 .... 61(03)
Carcinoid syndrome – 4848145 .... 61(07)
Cardiospasm – 4895132 – see Achalasia of cardia .... 61(11)
Cholecystitis, acute –
4154382 – see Chpt 22: Surgical Diseases .... 61(13)
Cholecystitis, chronic – 5481245 .... 61(16)
Cholecystolithiasis –
0148012 – see Chpt 22: Surgical Diseases .... 61(19)
Cirrhosis of the liver – 4812345 .... 61(22)
Cirrhosis, pigment – 5454589 – see Hemochromatosis .... 61(27)
Colitis – 8454321 .... 61(30)
Colitis, acute – 5432145 .... 61(32)
Colitis, chronic – 5481238 .... 62(01)
Constipation – 5484548 .... 62(05)
Diarrhea – 5843218 .... 62(08)
Diarrhea, functional –
81234574 – see Dyskinesia of the digestive tract .... 62(14)
Duodenal stasis –
8123457 – see Dyskinesia of the digestive tract .... 62(17)
Duodenitis – 5432114 .... 62(20)
Duodenitis, acute – 481543288 .... 62(23)
Duodenitis, chronic – 8432154 .... 62(28)

Dysbiosis, intestinal (Dysbacteriosis, intestinal) –
5432101.. 62(33)
Dyskinesia of the digestive tract (Dyspepsia;
Gastroptosis; Diarrhea, functional) – 81234574.................... 63(01)
Dyskinesia, biliary – 58432144 .... 63(07)
Dyskinesia, intestines – 54321893...................................... 63(11)
Dyspepsia (Indigestion) – 1112223 .... 63(19)
Dyspepsia, functional (Hyperacidity, stomach) –
5484214.. 63(24)
Enteritis – 8431287.. 63(29)
Enteritis, chronic – 5432140... 63(32)
Enterocolitis – 8454321 – see Colitis; Enteritis..................... 64(01)
Enteropathy, disaccharidase deficiency
(Lactose intolerance, Sucrose intolerance) – 4845432 .... 64(03)
Enteropathy, exudative – 48123454....................................... 64(08)
Enteropathy, gluten-induced (Celiac sprue;
Nontropical sprue; Steatorrhea, idiopathic) – 4891483 .... 64(12)
Enteropathy, of the intestines – 8432150................................ 64(19)
Esophagism – 5481248... 64(24)
Esophagitis – 54321489... 64(30)
Esophagospasm – 8123457 – see Dyskinesia of
the digestive tract and Esophagus spasm............................. 64(34)
Esophagus, peptic ulcer – 8432182 .... 65(01)
Food allergy – 2841482 .... 65(05)
Gastritis – 5485674.. 65(09)
Gastritis, acute – 4567891... 65(13)
Gastritis, chronic – 5489120 .... 65(19)
Gastrocardial syndrome (Roemheld syndrome) –
5458914.. 65(23)
Gastroenteritis – 5485674 – see Gastritis, Enteritis................ 65(29)
Gastroenterocolitis – 5485674 – see Gastritis, Enteritis.......... 65(31)
Gastrointestinal tuberculosis – 8143215................................ 65(34)
Gastroparesis (Gastric atony, acute) – 5485671 .... 66(03)
Gastroptosis –
81234574 – see Dyskinesia of the digestive tract.................. 66(08)
Hemochromatosis (Pigment cirrhosis, Bronze diabetes,
Iron overload disease, Siderophilia, Troisier-Hanot-
Chauffard syndrome) – 5454589 .... 66(11)
Hepatic insufficiency (Liver failure) – 8143214..................... 66(18)

Hepatitis – 5814243 .... 66(22)
Hepatitis, acute – 58432141 .... 66(24)
Hepatitis, chronic – 5123891 .... 66(31)
Hepatolenticular degeneration
(Wilson-Konowalow disease) – 5438912 .... 67(01)
Hepatosis – 9876512 .... 67(06)
Hepatosis, acute (Liver damage, toxic) – 1234576 .... 67(11)
Hepatosis, cholestatic (Cholestasis) – 5421548 .... 67(15)
Hepatosis, chronic – 5143214 .... 67(20)
Hepatosplenomegalic lipoidosis –
4851888 – see Hyperlipidemia .... 67(24)
Hepatosplenomegaly syndrome
(Hepatolienalic syndrome)– 8451485 .... 67(27)
Hyperbilirubinemia, benign – 84514851 .... 67(31)
Hyperbilirubinemia, congenital – 8432180 .... 68(03)
Hyperbilirubinemia, posthepatic
(Obstructive jaundice) – 8214321 .... 68(07)
Hyperlipidemia, idiopathic (Hyperliproteinemia,
Hepatosplenomegalic lipoidosis) – 4851888 .... 68(12)
Hypovitaminosis – 5154231 – see Chpt 15:
Diseases from a Lack of Vitamins .... 68(17)
Ileitis – 8431287 – see Enteritis .... 68(20)
Ileocecal valve inflammation (Bauhinitis) – 58432148 .... 68(22)
Indigestion – 9988771 .... 68(25)
Insufficiency of the cardiac sphincter – 8545142 .... 68(29)
Jaundice (Icterus) – 5432148 .... 68(34)
Jaundice, functional –
84514851 – see Hyperbilirubinemia, functional .... 69(05)
Jejunitis – 8431287 – see Enteritis .... 69(08)
Lipodystrophy, intestinal (Whipple's disease) –
4814548 .... 69(10)
Liver dystrophy – 9876512 – see Hepatosis .... 69(15)
Lymphangiectasia of the colon –
5214321 – see also Enteropathy of the colon .... 69(17)
Malabsorption – 48543215 .... 69(20)
Pancreatitis, acute – 4881431 – see Chpt 22:
Surgical Diseases .... 69(24)
Pancreatitis, chronic – 5891432 .... 69(27)
Peptic ulcer disease of the stomach and duodenum –

8125432.. 69(31)
Pneumatosis, gastric – 54321455.. 70(01)
Portal hypertension – 8143218 .... 70(04)
Post-hepatitis syndrome – 4812819...................................... 70(08)
Scurvy – 5432190 .... 70(14)
Spasm, intestinal (Colic, intestinal) –
8123457 – see Dyskinesia of the digestive tract..................... 70(17)
Sprue, nontropical –
8432150 – see Enteropathy, of the intestines......................... 70(20)
Sprue, tropical (Diarrhea, tropical) – 5481215 .... 70(23)
Starvation edema (Hunger edema, Famine dropsy,
Alimentary dystrophy) – 5456784....................................... 70(29)
Stomach phlegmon – 4567891 – see Gastritis, acute .... 71(01)
Stomach ulcers, symptomatic – 9671428 .... 71(04)
Superior mesenteric artery (SMA) syndrome –
5891234.. 71(08)
Ulcer of the small intestine, simple nonspecific –
48481452.. 71(13)
Whipple's disease –
4814548 – see Lipodystrophy, intestinal .... 71(19)
Zinga – 54321481 – see Chpt 15:
Diseases from a Lack of Vitamins: Vitamin C deficiency ...... 71(22)

**Chapter 9   DISEASES OF THE KIDNEYS AND
            URINARY TRACT – 8941254................... 72(07)**
Amyloidosis – 4512345 .... 72(11)
Cystitis – 48543211 .... 72(16)
Glomerulonephritis (diffuse proliferative GN) – 4812351 ..... 72(19)
Glomerulonephritis, acute – 4285614.................................. 72(23)
Hydronephrosis – 5432154.. 72(25)
Kidney disease, chronic (Kidney failure, chronic) –
5488821.. 72(30)
Nephrolithiasis (Kidney stones) – 5432143.......................... 72(33)
Polycystic kidney disease (PKD) – 5421451......................... 73(01)
Prostrate adenoma – 51432144 – See Chpt 22:
Surgical Diseases, Prostrate adenoma................................... 73(05)
Pyelitis – 5432110... 73(08)
Pyelonephritis – 58143213 .... 73(10)
Renal colic – 4321054 .... 73(14)

Renal Eclampsia – 8149141 – see also Glomerulonephritis, acute and Chpt 17: Obstetrics, Toxemia, in pregnancy (Pre-eclampsia) .... 73(18)
Renal failure (Kidney failure) – 4321843 .... 73(22)
Renal failure, acute (Kidney failure, acute) – 8218882 .... 73(28)
Renal insufficiency – 4321843 – see Renal failure .... 73(31)
Renal tuberculosis (Tuberculosis of the kidney) – 5814543 ... 73(33)
Uremia, acute – 5421822 – see also Renal failure, acute .... 74(01)
Uremia, chronic –
8914381 – see also Kidney disease, chronic .... 74(04)
Urethritis – 1387549 .... 74(07)
Urinary system, anomalies – 1234571 .... 74(10)

Chapter 10 BLOOD DISEASES – 1843214 .... 75(07)
Agranulocytosis – 4856742 .... 75(10)
Anemia – 48543212 .... 75(14)
Anemia, from lead poisoning – 1237819 .... 75(17)
Anemia, aplastic (hypoplastic) – 5481541 .... 75(21)
Anemia, autoimmune hemolytic – 5814311 .... 75(27)
Anemia, congenital; disruption of the synthesis of porphyrine – 4581254 .... 75(31)
Anemia, hemolytic – 5484813 .... 76(03)
Anemia, megaloblastic – 5481254 .... 76(06)
Anemia, posthemorrhagic acute (Blood loss, acute) – 9481232 .... 76(11)
Anemia, sickle-cell – 7891017 .... 76(15)
Chemotherapy, side effects of – 4812813 .... 76(20)
Favism – 54321457 .... 76(26)
Gaucher's disease (Cerebroside lipoidosis) – 5145432 .... 76(31)
Hemoblastosis outside of bone marrow, Hematosarcoma, and Lymphoma (Lymphocytoma) – 54321451 .... 77(01)
Hemorrhagic diathesis – 5148543 .... 77(08)
Hemorrhagic diathesis, caused by a pathology of the blood vessels – 54815438 .... 77(11)
Hypoprothrombinemia – 5481542 .... 77(16)
Leukemia – 5481347 .... 77(20)
Leukemoid reactions – 5814321 .... 77(24)
Lymphogranulomatosis (Hodgkin's lymphoma) – 4845714 .. 77(31)
Myelocytosis (Leukemia, chronic myeloid) – 5142357 .... 78(01)

Neutropenia, congenital – 8432145 .... 78(04)
Ovalocytosis, hereditary (Elliptocytosis, hereditary) –
51454323.. 78(09)
Paraproteinemia producing tumors – 8432184 .... 78(14)
Paroxysmal nocturnal hemoglobinuria (PNH) – 5481455...... 78(20)
Radiation sickness, acute – 481543294 .... 78(26)
Radiation sickness, chronic – 4812453................................ 78(31)
Stomatocytosis, hereditary – 4814581 .... 79(01)
Thalassemia – 7765437... 79(05)
Thrombocytopathy – 5418541 .... 79(10)
Thrombophilia, hematogenous – 4814543 .... 79(14)

Chapter 11   ENDOCRINE AND METABOLIC
               DISORDERS – 1823451............................80(07)
Acromegaly – 1854321.. 80(10)
Addison's disease (Adrenal insufficiency) – 4812314........... 80(15)
Cushing's syndrome – 54321458.. 80(21)
Diabetes insipidus – 4818888 .... 80(25)
Diabetes mellitus – 8819977.. 80(30)
Puberal juvenile dyspituitarism syndrome – 4145412........... 81(01)
Gender differentiation, congenital disorders of –
5451432.. 81(07)
Goiter, endemic – 5432178.. 81(11)
Goiter, toxic diffuse (Graves' Disease) – 5143218................ 81(15)
Growth hormone deficiency (Hypophyseal dwarfism) –
4141414.. 81(19)
Hyperinsulinemia (Dysinsulinism) – 48454322 .... 81(23)
Hyperprolactinemia – 4812454.. 81(29)
Hypogonadism (male) – 48143121....................................... 81(33)
Hypoparathyroidism (Parathyroid tetany) – 4514321 .... 82(01)
Hypopituitarism (Panhypopituitarism,
Simmond's disease) – 48143214 .... 82(06)
Hypothyroidism (Myxedema) – 4812415.............................. 82(11)
Obesity – 4812412... 82(14)
Osteitis fibrosa cystica – 5481412 .... 82(17)
Pheochromocytoma – 4818145.. 82(21)
Sexual development, premature – 4814312........................... 82(26)
Thyroiditis – 4811111 .... 82(30)
Tumors (see also: Acromegaly, Virilism, Hyperinsulinemia,

Hyperparathyroidism, Pheochromocytoma) – 4541548 .... 82(34)

Virilism – 89143212 .... 83(04)

Chapter 12 OCCUPATIONAL DISEASES –
4185481 ....84(07)

Occupational diseases, caused by chemical agents –
9916515 .... 84(10)

Occupational diseases, exposure to physical factors
(Vibration disease) – 4514541 .... 84(14)

Occupational diseases, through the influence of
biological agents – 81432184 .... 84(19)

Occupational diseases, through overexertion – 4814542 .... 84(23)

Chapter 13 ACUTE TOXICATION – 4185412 ....85(07)

Acute poisonings: percutaneous – 4814823 .... 85(10)

Acute poisonings: ingestion – 5142154 .... 85(13)

Acute poisonings: inhalation – 4548142 .... 85(17)

Acute poisonings: injected – 4818142 .... 85(20)

Acute poisonings: snakebites, other
poisonous arthropods – 4812521 .... 85(24)

Acute poisonings: scorpion stings – 4188888 .... 85(28)

Acute poisonings: snakebites – 4114111 .... 85(32)

Acute poisonings: tarantula spider bites – 8181818 .... 86(01)

Acute poisonings: wasp and bee stings – 9189189 .... 86(06)

Exotoxic shock – 4185421 .... 86(10)

Kidney damage (Toxic nephropathy) – 5412123 .... 86(14)

Liver damage (Hepatopathy, toxic) – 48145428 .... 86(19)

Psychoneurotic disorder from toxic exposure – 9977881 .... 86(25)

Chapter 14 INFECTIOUS DISEASES –
5421427 ....87(07)

Alveolococcosis (Alveolar echinococcosis,
Small fox tapeworm) – 5481454 .... 87(10)

Amoebiasis – 1289145 .... 87(14)

Ankylostomiasis (Hookworm infestation) – 4815454 .... 87(20)

Anthrax – 9998991 .... 87(24)

Ascariasis – 4814812 .... 87(27)

Balantidiasis – 1543218 .... 87(31)

Botkin's disease – 5412514 – see also Hepatitis,

viral A and B .... 88(01)
Botulism, foodborne – 5481252 .... 88(04)
Brill-Zinsser disease – 514854299 .... 88(07)
Brucellosis (Bang's disease, Malta fever) – 4122222 .... 88(10)
Campylobacter jejuni – 4815421 .... 88(14)
Cat scratch disease (Lymphadenitis, subacute regional) –
48145421 .... 88(18)
Cholera – 4891491 .... 88(22)
Clonorchiasis (Chinese liver fluke) – 5412348 .... 88(25)
Cysticercosis – 4512824 .... 88(29)
Diphtheria – 5556679 .... 89(01)
Diphyllobothriasis (Fish or broad tapeworm infestation) –
4812354 .... 89(07)
Dysentery (Shigellosis) – 4812148 .... 89(11)
E. coli bacteriosis (Escherichiosis) – 1238888 .... 89(15)
Echinococcosis – 5481235 .... 89(20)
Encephalitis, tick-borne – 7891010 .... 89(24)
Enterobiasis – 5123542 .... 89(29)
Enteroviruses – 8123456 .... 89(33)
Erysipelas – 4123548 .... 90(04)
Fascioliosis (Fascioliasis) – 4812542 .... 90(09)
Food poisoning – 5184231 .... 90(13)
Foot and mouth disease – 9912399 .... 90(18)
Giardiasis (Lambliasis) – 5189148 .... 90(23)
Helminthiasis – 5124548 .... 90(28)
Hemorrhagic fever with renal syndrome – 5124567 .... 90(32)
Hepatitis, viral, A und B (Botkin's disease) – 5412514 .... 91(01)
Herpes simplex – 2312489 .... 91(08)
Human immunodeficiency virus (HIV, AIDS) – 5148555 ...... 91(13)
Hydrophobia – 4812543 – see Rabies .... 91(19)
Hymenolepiasis (Dwarf tapeworm infestation) – 54812548 .. 91(21)
Influenza, seasonal (Flu) – 4814212 .... 91(24)
Legionellosis (Legionnaires' disease) – 5142122 .... 91(27)
Leishmaniasis – 5184321 .... 91(33)
Leprosy – 148543294 – see Chpt 21:
Skin and Venereal Diseases, Leprosy .... 92(01)
Leptospirosis (Canicola fever, Weil's disease) – 5128432 ..... 92(04)
Listeriosis – 5812438 .... 92(08)
Lyssa – 4812543 – see Rabies .... 92(12)

© Г. П. Грабовой, 1999

Malaria – 5189999 .... 92(14)
Marburg virus disease (Marburg hemorrhagic fever,
Ebola) – 5184599 .... 92(18)
Meningococcal infection – 5891423 .... 92(24)
Metagonimiasis – 54812541 .... 92(29)
Mononucleosis, infectious (Pfeiffer's disease,
Kissing disease) – 5142548 .... 92(34)
Mycoplasma infection (Pneumonia, atypical;
Pneumonia, walking) – 5481111 .... 93(05)
Opisthorchiasis – 5124542 .... 93(11)
Ornithosis (Psittacosis) – 5812435 .... 93(15)
Parapertussis – 2222221 .... 93(19)
Parotitis epidemica (Mumps) – 3218421 .... 93(23)
Pediculosis (Lice, infestation of) – 48148121 .... 93(28)
Pertussis (Whooping cough) – 4812548 .... 93(32)
Plague – 8998888 .... 94(01)
Q-Fever – 5148542 .... 94(04)
Rabies (Hydrophobia, Lyssa) – 4812543 .... 94(08)
Rotavirus – 5148567 .... 94(11)
Rubella (German measles) – 4218547 .... 94(14)
Rubeola (Measles) – 4214825 .... 94(19)
Salmonellosis – 5142189 .... 94(24)
Scarlatina (Scarlet fever) – 5142485 .... 94(27)
Schistosomiasis (Bilharziosis) – 48125428 .... 94(33)
Strongyloidiasis – 54812527 .... 95(04)
Taeniarhynchosis – 4514444 .... 95(09)
Taeniasis – 4855555 .... 95(12)
Tetanus (Lockjaw) – 5671454 .... 95(17)
Toxoplasmosis – 8914755 .... 95(22)
Trichinellosis – 7777778 .... 95(26)
Trichocephalosis (Trichuriasis) – 4125432 .... 95(29)
Trichostrongylosis – 9998888 .... 95(33)
Tularemia – 4819489 .... 96(01)
Typhoid and paratyphoid fever (Abdominal typhus)–
1411111 .... 96(04)
Typhus, epidemic – 1444444 .... 96(10)
Typhus, Queensland tick typhus (Spotted fever)–
5189499 .... 96(15)
Upper respiratory tract infection (Common cold) –

48145488 .... 96(20)
Varicella (Chickenpox) – 48154215 .... 96(25)
Variola (Smallpox) – 4848148 .... 96(30)
Variola minor – 4848148 .... 97(01)
Yersinia pseudotuberculosis – 514854212 .... 97(04)
Yersiniosis – 5123851 .... 97(09)

**Chapter 15 VITAMIN DEFICIENCY
DISEASES – 1234895 .... 98(07)**
Avitaminosis – 5451234 .... 98(10)
Hypovitaminosis – 5154231 .... 98(15)
Polyavitaminosis – 4815432 .... 98(20)
Vitamin A deficiency (Retinol deficiency) – 4154812 .... 98(23)
Vitamin B1 deficiency (Thiamine deficiency) – 1234578 ...... 98(28)
Vitamin B2 deficiency (Riboflavin deficiency) – 1485421 ..... 99(01)
Vitamin B3 deficiency (Vitamin PP deficiency,
Niacin deficiency) – 1842157 .... 99(06)
Vitamin B6 deficiency (Pyridoxine deficiency) – 9785621 .... 99(13)
Vitamin C deficiency (Ascorbic acid deficiency) –
4141255 .... 99(21)
Vitamin D deficiency – 5421432 .... 99(24)
Vitamin K deficiency – 4845414 .... 99(28)

**Chapter 16 DISEASES IN CHILDHOOD -
18543218 .... 100(07)**
Adrenal hyperplasia, congenital – 45143213 .... 100(10)
Allergic diathesis (Predisposition to allergies) – 0195451 ..... 100(14)
Allergies, respiratory – 45143212 .... 100(18)
Alpha 1-antitrypsin deficiency – 1454545 .... 100(22)
Anemia – 48543212 – see Chpt 10: Blood Diseases .... 100(26)
Anemia, iron deficiency – 1458421 .... 100(28)
Anemia, toxic hemolytic – 45481424 .... 100(33)
Asthma bronchiale – 58145428 .... 101(01)
Bronchitis, acute – 5482145 .... 101(06)
Bronchitis, allergic – 5481432 .... 101(09)
Celiac disease – 4154548 .... 101(15)
Cramps (Spasms) – 51245424 .... 101(18)
Cystic fibrosis (Mucoviscidosis) – 9154321 .... 101(22)
De Toni–Debré–Fankoni syndrome – 4514848 .... 101(28)

Diabetes insipidus – 5121111 .... 101(34)
Diabetes mellitus – 4851421 .... 102(04)
Diabetes, phosphate – 5148432 .... 102(10)
Dyspepsia, parenteral – 8124321 .... 102(15)
Dyspepsia, simple – 5142188 .... 102(20)
Dyspepsia, toxic – 514218821 .... 102(27)
Dystonia, vegetative-circulatory – 514218838 .... 102(31)
Exudative enteropathy (Enteropathy, protein-losing) –
4548123 .... 103(01)
Fetal alcohol syndrome – 4845421 .... 103(07)
Foreign object aspiration – 4821543 .... 103(12)
Galactosemia – 48125421 .... 103(16)
Glomerulonephritis, in children – 5145488 .... 103(20)
Heart defect, congenital (childhood) – 14891548 .... 103(23)
Hemolytic disease of the newborn (Rhesus disease,
Erythroblastosis fetalis) – 5125432 .... 103(30)
Hemophilia – 548214514 .... 104(01)
Hemorrhagic diathesis – 0480421 –
see also Purpura rheumatica, Hemophilia .... 104(04)
Hemorrhagic disease of the newborn – 5128543 .... 104(07)
Hepatitis – see Chpt 8: Disorders of the Digestive Organs .... 104(10)
Histiocytosis, x-type – 5484321 .... 104(13)
Hypervitaminosis D – 5148547 .... 104(17)
Hypothyroidism – 4512333 .... 104(21)
Infantile tetany (Spasmophilia) – 5148999 .... 104(24)
Intracranial birth trauma – 518999981 .... 104(29)
Jaundice, neonatal (Icterus neonatorum) – 4815457 .... 104(33)
Laryngitis, allergic – 58143214 .... 105(01)
Leukemia – 5481347 – see Chpt 10: Blood Diseases .... 105(06)
Lymphatic predisposition – 5148548 .... 105(08)
Malabsorption syndrome – 4518999 .... 105(13)
Nephritis, hereditary (Alport syndrome) – 5854312 .... 105(18)
Phenylketonuria – 5148321 .... 105(23)
Pneumonia, chronic – 51421543 .... 105(27)
Pneumonia, interstitial – 4814489 – see Chpt 7:
Respiratory Diseases, Pneumonia .... 105(32)
Pneumonia, neonatal – 5151421 .... 106(01)

Pneumonitis, hypersensitive (Allergic alveolitis) –

51843215.. 106(04)
Polyarthritis, chronic unspecified – 8914201 – see Chpt 6:
Rheumatic Diseases, Arthritis, rheumatoid........................... 106(08)
Portal Hypertension – 45143211.. 106(11)
Pseudocroup – 5148523.. 106(17)
Pseudocroup (Laryngitis, subglottic;
Laryngotracheobronchitis) – 1489542.............................. 106(19)
Purpura rheumatica (Henoch-Schoenlein purpura,
Schoenlein-Henoch purpura) – 5128421 .... 106(24)
Pyloric stenosis (Infantile hypertrophic pyloric stenosis) –
5154321 – see Chpt 22: Surgeries, Surgeries on infants........ 106(30)
Pylorospasm – 5141482.. 106(34)
Renal diabetes (Renal glucosuria) – 5142585 .... 107(03)
Renal salt-wasting syndrome
(Pseudohypoaldosteronism) – 3245678.............................. 107(07)
Respiratory distress syndrome in newborns – 5148284 .... 107(13)
Rheumatism – 5481543 .... 107(18)
Rhinitis und Sinusitis, allergic – 5814325 .... 107(21)
Rickets (Vitamin D deficiency, Rachitis) – 5481232............. 107(27)
Sepsis, neonatorum – 4514821 .... 107(32)
Staphylococcus infection – 5189542 .... 108(01)
Subfebrile condition in children – 5128514........................ 108(05)
Subsepsis allergica (Wissler's syndrome) – 5421238............ 108(10)
Toxic syndrome (Toxicosis with exsiccosis) – 5148256 .... 108(14)
Tracheitis, allergic – 514854218....................................... 108(19)
Tuberculosis – 5148214.. 108(23)
Tuberculosis, latent (Tuberculosis, asymptomatic) –
1284345.. 108(27)
Vomiting – 1454215.. 108(32)

***Surgical Conditions in Children* – 5182314**...................**109(06)**
Angioma (Hemangioma) – 4812599 .... 109(12)
Appendicitis, childhood – 9999911 .... 109(15)
Atresia and stenosis, duodenal – 5557777.......................... 109(19)
Atresia, anal and rectal – 6555557.................................... 109(22)
Atresia, biliary – 9191918... 109(25)
Atresia, esophageal – 8194321 .... 109(28)
Atresia, small intestine – 9188888.................................... 109(31)
Cephalohematoma (Subperiostal hemorrhage) –

48543214.. 109(34)

Esophagus, chemical burn of – 5148599 .... 110(04)

Hemorrhage, gastrointestinal – 5121432 .... 110(07)

Hernia, diaphragmatic – 5189412 .... 110(11)

Invagination – 5148231 .... 110(17)

Meckel's diverticulum – 4815475 .... 110(21)

Omphalocele (Amniocele) – 5143248 .... 110(25)

Osteomyelitis, epiphyseal – 12345895 .... 110(30)

Palatoschisis (Cleft palate) – 5151515 .... 110(33)

Phlegmon, newborns – 51485433 .... 111(01)

Pyloric stenosis – 5154321 .... 111(05)

Teratoma, sacrococcygeal region – 481543238 .... 111(10)

Chapter 17 OBSTETRICS, GYNECOLOGICAL
DISORDERS – 1489145 .... 112(07)

Amniotic fluid embolism – 5123412 .... 112(11)

Asphyxia, perinatal – 4812348 .... 112(16)

Hemorrhage, during childbirth – 4814821 .... 112(20)

Labor, abnormal patterns during – 14891543 .... 112(24)

Milk glands, dysfunction of during lactation period –
48123147 .... 112(29)

Mole, hydatidiform – 4121543 .... 112(33)

Pain management during childbirth – 5421555 .... 113(01)

Pelvis, narrow – 2148543 .... 113(07)

Pelvis, narrow (anatomically) – 4812312 .... 113(11)

Pelvis, narrow (clinically) – 4858543 .... 113(15)

Placenta praevia – 1481855 .... 113(21)

Placental abruption – 1111155 .... 113(25)

Polyhydramnios (Hydramnios) – 5123481 .... 113(33)

Postnatal/postpartum period, normal – 12891451 .... 114(01)

Postpartum complications – 41854218 .... 114(04)

Pregnancy, birth and due date – 1888711 .... 114(09)

Pregnancy, ectopic (for the restoration of health and
retention of the fetus) – 4812311 .... 114(16)

Pregnancy, multiple (pregnancy with two or more fetuses) –
123457854 .... 114(21)

Pregnancy, post-term (prolonged) – 5142148 .... 114(24)

Pregnancy, uterine – 1899911 .... 114(27)

Preterm birth – 1284321 .... 114(31)

Tears in external genitals during childbirth – 148543291 ...... 114(34)
Toxemia, in pregnancy (Pre-eclampsia) – 1848542 .... 115(04)
Umbilical cord wound care for newborns – 0123455............. 115(11)
Umbilical cord, prolapse – 1485432...................................... 115(17)
***Gynecological Disorders* – 1854312 ....115(22)**
Adnexitis – see Oophoritis, Salpingitis................... 115(24)
Adrenogenital syndrome – 148542121................. 115(26)
Amenorrhea – 514354832.................................... 115(30)
Anovulatory cycle – 4813542............................... 115(33)
Bartholinitis – 58143215...................................... 116(01)
Cancer, vulva – 5148945 .... 116(04)
Cervical erosion (Ectropion, cervical) – 54321459 .... 116(07)
Chorionepithelioma (Choriocarcinoma) – 4854123 .... 116(11)
Colpitis – 5148533.. 116(15)
Cyst, ovarian – 5148538 .... 116(17)
Cystadenoma, ovarian – 58432143....................... 116(20)
Dysmenorrhea – 4815812..................................... 116(23)
Endocervicitis – 4857148 .... 116(26)
Endometriosis – 5481489 .... 116(30)
Endometritis – 8142522.. 116(33)
Gonorrhea – 5148314 .... 117(01)
Hemorrhage, dysfunctional bleeding of the uterus –
4853541.. 117(04)
Infertility (Sterility) – 9918755............................. 117(09)
Kraurosis vulvae – 58143218 .... 117(13)
Leukoplakia, vulva or cervix – 5185321 .... 117(17)
Leukorrhea (Vaginal discharge) – 5128999........... 117(23)
Menopause (Climacteric) – 4851548..................... 117(27)
Myoma, uterine – 51843216.................................. 117(31)
Oophoritis (Adnexitis) – 5143548 .... 117(34)
Ovarian apoplexy (Corpus luteum rupture) – 1238543 .... 118(03)
Parametritis – 5143215 .... 118(08)
Polycystic Ovarian Disease (Stein-Leventhal syndrome) –
518543248.. 118(11)
Polyp, cervical or uterine – 518999973 .... 118(16)
Premenstrual syndrome (PMS) – 9917891 .... 118(20)
Prolapse, uterus and vagina – 514832183.............. 118(25)
Pruritus vulvae (Vulva, itchy) – 5414845 .... 118(30)
Salpingitis – 5148914 .... 118(33)

Tuberculosis, genital – 8431485 .... 119(01)
Vaginitis (Colpitis) – 5148533 .... 119(06)
Vulvitis – 5185432 .... 119(09)
Vulvovaginitis – 5814513 .... 119(12)

Chapter 18   NEUROLOGICAL DISEASES –
148543293 .... 120(07)
Abscess, cerebral – 1894811 .... 120(10)
Adie syndrome (Mydriasis, Pupillotonia) – 18543211 .... 120(13)
Amyotrophic lateral sclerosis (Motor neuron disease,
Lou Gehrig's disease) – 5148910 .... 120(17)
Aneurysm, cerebral – 1485999 .... 120(23)
Arachnoiditis – 4567549 .... 120(28)
Asthenia (Chronic fatigue syndrome) – 1891013 .... 120(32)
Athetosis – 1454891 .... 121(01)
Brain injury, traumatic – 51843213 .... 121(04)
Cerebral palsy – 4818521 .... 121(08)
Charcot-Marie-Tooth disease – 4814512 .... 121(13)
Chorea – 4831485 .... 121(18)
Coma – 1111012 .... 121(22)
Diencephalic syndrome (Hypothalamic syndrome) –
514854215 .... 121(25)
Encephalitis, viral – 48188884 .... 121(29)
Epiduritis – 888888149 .... 121(32)
Epilepsy – 1484855 .... 122(01)
Funicular myelitis (Putnam-Dana syndrome) –
518543251 .... 122(05)
Headache (Cephalgia) – 4818543 .... 122(10)
Headache, cluster – 4851485 .... 122(13)
Hepatocerebral dystrophy (Wilson's disease,
Hepatolenticular degeneration)– 48143212 .... 122(17)
Herpes zoster (Shingles) – 51454322 .... 122(24)
Hydrocephalus – 81432143 .... 122(28)
Meningitis – 51485431 .... 122(33)
Migraine – 4831421 .... 123(01)
Mononeuropathy – 4541421 .... 123(04)
Multiple Sclerosis – 51843218 .... 123(07)
Muscular dystrophy, progressive – 85432183 .... 123(12)
Myasthenia gravis – 9987542 .... 123(16)

Myelitis – 4891543 .... 123(20)
Myelopathia – 51843219 .... 123(24)
Myotonia congenita (Thomsen's disease) – 4848514 .... 123(28)
Myotonic dystrophy (Curschmann-Batten-Steiner
syndrome) – 481543244 .... 123(33)
Narcolepsy – 48543216 .... 124(05)
Neuropathy, facial nerves – 518999955 .... 124(10)
Neurorheumatism – 8185432 .... 124(14)
Neurosyphilis – 5482148 .... 124(17)
Ophthalmoplegia – 4848532 .... 124(21)
Paralysis, familial periodic – 5123488 .... 124(25)
Parkinson's disease (Parkinsonism) – 54811421 .... 124(29)
Phakomatoses – 5142314 .... 125(01)
Poliomyelitis (Paralysis, infantile) – 2223214 .... 125(05)
Polyneuropathy – 4838514 .... 125(11)
Polyneuropathy, acute inflammatory demyelinating
(Guillain-Barré syndrome) – 4548128 .... 125(16)
Post-lumbar puncture syndrome – 818543231 .... 125(21)
Radiculopathy (Radiculitis, Sciatica) – 5481321 .... 125(25)
Sleep disorder – 514248538 .... 125(30)
Spinal amyotrophy – 5483312 .... 125(34)
Spinal apoplexy (Spinal insult) – 8888881 .... 126(04)
Stroke (Apoplexy, Cerebrovascular insult, Spinal stroke
syndrome) – 4818542 .... 126(07)
Syncope (Fainting spells) – 4854548 .... 126(11)
Syringomyelia – 1777771 .... 126(16)
Tremor – 3148567 .... 126(21)
Trigeminal neuralgia – 5148485 .... 126(25)
Tumor, brain – 5451214 .... 126(29)
Tumor, brain and spinal cord – 5431547 – See Chpt 2:
Tumors, Tumor, brain and spinal cord .... 126(32)
Tumor, peripheral nervous system – 514832182 .... 127(01)
Tumor, spinal cord – 51843210 .... 127(05)
Vertigo, cerebral (Dizziness) – 514854217 .... 127(09)

**Chapter 19 PSYCHIATRIC DISORDERS –
                8345444 ....128(07)**
Affective disorder – 548142182 .... 128(10)
Alcoholism – 148543292 .... 128(17)

Bipolar disorder (Manic-depressive disorder) – 514218857 .. 128(24)
Catatonia – 51843214 .... 128(29)
Delusional disorder – 8142351 .... 128(33)
Encephalopathy, post-traumatic – 18543217 .... 129(01)
Grandiosity – 148454283 .... 129(06)
Hallucinosis – 4815428 .... 129(10)
Hypochondria – 1488588 .... 129(15)
Hysterical syndrome – 5154891 .... 129(19)
Korsakoff's syndrome – 4185432 .... 129(23)
Mental confusion – 4518533 .... 129(27)
Narcomania (Addiction to narcotics) – 5333353 ...... 129(32)
Narcomania and Toxicomania – 1414551 .... 130(06)
Negative (deficit) symptoms – 5418538 .... 130(10)
Neurotic disorder – 48154211 .... 130(15)
Obsessive compulsive disorder (Fixed ideas) – 8142543 .... 130(19)
Oligophrenia (Mental retardation) – 1857422 .... 130(23)
Paralysis, progressive – 512143223 .... 130(27)
Psychic defect – 8885512 .... 130(31)
Psychoorganic syndrome – 51843212 .... 131(01)
Psychopathic disorder (Antisocial personality disorder) –
4182546 .... 131(04)
Psychoses, symptomatic – 8148581 .... 131(09)
Psychosis, presenile (Psychosis, involutional) – 18543219 .... 131(14)
Psychosis, reactive – 0101255 .... 131(20)
Psychosis, senile – 481854383 .... 131(24)
Psychotic disorder, substance-induced – 1142351 ... 131(28)
Schizophrenia – 1858541 .... 131(33)

Chapter 20 SEXUAL DISORDERS – 1456891 .... 132(07)
Ejaculation disorders – 1482541 .... 132(10)
Erectile dysfunction – 184854281 .... 132(14)
Frigidity, female – 5148222 .... 132(19)
Hypersexuality – 5414855 .... 132(22)
Impotence – 8851464 .... 132(25)
Onanism (Masturbation) – 0021421 .... 132(28)
Psychosexual disorder (Sexual perversion) – 0001112 .... 132(31)
Sexual dysfunction – 1818191 .... 133(01)
Sexual dysfunction, from neuroendocrine disorders .... 133(06)
Sexual dysfunction, imaginary – 1484811 .... 133(11)

Sexual dysfunction, psychic – 2148222 .... 133(16)
Vaginismus – 5142388 .... 133(20)

Chapter 21 DERMATOLOGICAL AND
VENEREAL DISEASES – 18584321 .... 134(07)
Acne vulgaris – 514832185 .... 134(11)
Actinomycosis of the skin – 148542156 .... 134(15)
Alopecia (Baldness, Hair loss) – 5484121 .... 134(18)
Balanoposthitis – 5814231 .... 134(22)
Candidiasis (Thrush, Yeast infection) – 9876591 .... 134(25)
Condyloma acuminatum (Fig warts, Genital warts) –
1489543 .... 134(30)
Dermatitis – 1853121 .... 135(01)
Dermatitis, atopic (Neurodermitis, diffuse) – 5484215 .... 135(05)
Eczema – 548132151 .... 135(10)
Erythema multiforme – 548142137 .... 135(15)
Erythema nodosum – 15184321 .... 135(19)
Erythrasma – 4821521 .... 135(23)
Favus – 4851481 .... 135(26)
Gonorrhea, in men – 2225488 .... 135(30)
Gonorrhea, in women – 5148314 – see Chpt 17:
Obstetrics, Gynecological Disorders, Gonorrhea .... 135(34)
Ichthyosis – 9996789 .... 136(01)
Leprosy – 148543294 .... 136(04)
Leukoderma (Vitiligo) – 4812588 .... 136(06)
Lichen ruber planus – 4858415 .... 136(11)
Lyell's syndrome (Epidermal necrolyses, toxic) – 4891521 ... 136(15)
Lymphogranulomatosis inguinalis – 1482348 .... 136(20)
Mastocytosis – 148542171 .... 136(23)
Molluscum contagiosum – 514321532 .... 136(26)
Mycosis fungoides – 4814588 .... 136(29)
Neurodermatitis – 1484857 .... 136(32)
Pemphigus (Blistering disease) – 8145321 .... 137(01)
Pityriasis rosea – 5148315 .... 137(06)
Pityriasis versicolor – 18543214 .... 137(09)
Prurigo nodularis – 5189123 .... 137(12)
Pruritus (Itching) – 1249812 .... 137(16)
Psoriasis – 999899181 .... 137(21)
Pyoderma – 51432149 .... 137(25)

Ringworm (Epidermophyton) – 5148532 .... 137(28)
Ringworm (Microsporum) – 1858321 .... 137(31)
Ringworm (Trichophytosis) – 4851482 .... 138(01)
Rosacea – 518914891 .... 138(04)
Scabies – 8132548 .... 138(09)
Seborrhea – 1234512 .... 138(13)
Skin toxicosis – 514832184 .... 138(17)
Steven-Johnson syndrome – 9814753 .... 138(22)
Syphilis (Lues) – 1484999 .... 138(27)
Trichophyton rubrum – 4518481 .... 138(31)
Tuberculosis, cutaneous – 148543296 .... 139(01)
Tumor, skin – 1458914 .... 139(05)
Ulcus molle (Chancroid, Soft Chancre) – 4815451 .... 139(08)
Urticaria (Hives) – 1858432 .... 139(12)
Vasculitides, cutaneous – 5142544 .... 139(16)
Vasculitis (Angiitis, cutaneous) – 1454231 .... 139(20)
Verrucae (Warts) – 5148521 .... 139(24)

Chapter 22 SURGICAL DISEASES – 18574321 .... 140(07)
Surgical Diseases in Adults – 5843215 .... 140(09)
Abdomen, acute – 5484543 .... 140(12)
Abscess – 8148321 .... 140(15)
Actinomycosis – 4832514 .... 140(18)
Anal fissure – 81454321 .... 140(22)
Aneurysm – 48543218 .... 140(26)
Appendicitis, acute – 54321484 .... 140(32)
Bronchiectasis – 4812578 .... 141(01)
Burns, thermal – 8191111 .... 141(05)
Carbuncle – 483854381 .... 141(09)
Cardiac aneurysm – 9187549 .... 141(12)
Cholangitis – 8431548 .... 141(15)
Cholecystitis, acute – 4154382 .... 141(18)
Cholecystolithiasis – 0148012 .... 141(21)
Colitis, ulcerative – 48143211 .... 141(25)
Contusion (Bruise) – 0156912 .... 141(30)
Crohn's disease – 94854321 .... 141(33)
Cryptorchidism – 485143287 .... 142(05)
Cyst, branchial cleft (Cyst, lateral neck,
Pharyngeal fistula) – 514854214 .... 142(08)

Cyst, breast (Fibrocystic breasts) – 4851432 .... 142(13)
Cyst, thyroglossal (Cyst, median neck) – 4548541 .... 142(17)
Decubitus (Bed sores) – 6743514 .... 142(21)
Diverticulosis, colon – 4851614 .... 142(27)
Diverticulum – 48543217 .... 142(33)
Dumping syndrome (gastric) – 4184214 .... 143(01)
Electric shock injuries – 5185431 .... 143(06)
Empyema, pleural (Pleuritis, purulent) – 514854223 .... 143(10)
Endangiitis obliterans – 4518521 .... 143(14)
Fibroadenoma, breast – 4854312 .... 143(19)
Fistula, epithelial coccygeal, (Cyst, pilonidal) – 9018532 ...... 143(22)
Fistula, rectal – 5189421 .... 143(28)
Flat feet (Pes planus, Platypodia) – 1891432 .... 143(34)
Foreign objects, bronchi – 5485432 .... 144(03)
Foreign objects, esophagus – 14854321 .... 144(07)
Foreign objects, soft tissue – 148543297 .... 144(11)
Foreign objects, stomach – 8184321 .... 144(15)
Fracture – 7776551 .... 144(19)
Frostbite – 4858514 .... 144(22)
Furuncle (Boil) – 5148385 .... 144(25)
Gas gangrene – 41543218 .... 144(28)
Gynecomastia – 4831514 .... 144(31)
Hemarthrosis – 4857543 .... 144(33)
Hemorrhage, external (Bleeding, external) – 4321511 .... 145(01)
Hemorrhage, internal (Bleeding, internal) – 5142543 .... 145(06)
Hemorrhoids – 58143219 .... 145(11)
Hernia – 95184321 .... 145(14)
Hidradenitis – 4851348 .... 145(17)
Hydrocele, testis or spermatic cord – 481543255 .... 145(22)
Ileus, paralytic (Intestinal stasis) – 4548148 .... 145(24)
Ingrown nail (Onychocryptosis) – 4548547 .... 145(28)
Jaundice, obstructive – 8012001 .... 145(32)
Leiomyoma – 55114214 .... 146(01)
Lipoma – 4814842 .... 146(04)
Luxation – 5123145 .... 146(07)
Lymphadenitis – 4542143 .... 146(09)
Lymphangitis – 484851482 .... 146(12)
Mastitis – 8152142 .... 146(15)
Mastopathy – 84854321 .... 146(18)

Mediastinitis – 4985432 .... 146(21)
Megacolon – 4851543 .... 146(25)
Meniscus tear – 8435482 .... 146(29)
Occlusion of major arteries – 81543213 .... 146(32)
Orchiepididymitis – 818432151 .... 147(01)
Osteomyelitis, traumatic – 514854221 .... 147(04)
Pancreatitis, acute – 4881431 .... 147(08)
Paronychia (Panaritium) – 8999999 .... 147(12)
Peritonitis – 1428543 .... 147(15)
Phimosis, Paraphimosis – 0180010 .... 147(20)
Phlebothrombosis – 1454580 .... 147(25)
Phlegmon – 48143128 .... 147(29)
Pneumothorax, spontaneous – 481854221 .... 147(32)
Polyp – 4819491 .... 148(01)
Postcholecystectomy syndrome – 4518421 .... 148(05)
Prostatitis – 9718961 .... 148(09)
Prostrate adenoma – 51432144 .... 148(12)
Pseudarthrosis – 4814214 .... 148(16)
Pulmonary gangrene – 4838543 .... 148(21)
Pyloric stenosis – 81543211 .... 148(25)
Pyopneumothorax – 148543299 .... 148(30)
Rectal prolapse – 514832187 .... 148(33)
Sebaceous cyst (Steatoma) – 888888179 .... 149(01)
Talipes equinovarus (Clubfoot) – 485143241 .... 149(04)
Thrombangiitis obliterans (Buerger's disease) – 5432142 ..... 149(08)
Thrombophlebitis – 1454580 – see Phlebothrombosis .... 149(14)
Torticollis (Wryneck) – 4548512 .... 149(16)
Trauma, inner organs – 8914319 .... 149(20)
Tuberculosis, bone – 148543281 .... 149(23)
Ulcer (stomach or duodenum), penetrating – 9148532 .... 149(26)
Ulcer, penetrating – 8143291 .... 149(30)
Ulcer, trophic – 514852154 .... 149(34)
Urinary retention, acute (Ischuria, acute) – 0144444 .... 150(03)
Varicocele – 81432151 .... 150(08)
Varicosis – 4831388 .... 150(12)
Wounds – 5148912 .... 150(16)
Zollinger-Ellison syndrome – 148543295 .... 150(19)
Surgical Diseases of the Newborn – 514218871 ..... ***150(23)***
Cholangiopathy of the newborn, congenital – 948514211 ..... 150(25)

Surgical diseases of organs of abdominal cavity – 5184311 .. 150(29)
Surgical Diseases of the Thorax Organs – 5184312 .... **151(01)**
Atresia, esophagus – 518543157 .... 151(03)
Cystic lung disease, congenital – 4851484 .... 151(08)
Fistula, tracheoesophageal – 514854714 .... 151(12)
Hernia, congenital diaphragmatic – 518543257 .... 151(17)
Pneumothorax – 5142147 .... 151(23)
Purulent Inflammatory Diseases – 514852171 .... **151(27)**
Mastitis, newborns – 514854238 .... 151(29)
Musculoskeletal system, diseases in newborns –
514218873 .... 151(32)
Osteomyelitis, acute hematogenous in newborns –
5141542 .... 152(01)
Paraproctitis, acute – 4842118 .... 152(04)
Peritonitis, newborns – 4184321 .... 152(08)
Phlegmon, necrotic cutaneous, in newborns – 514852173 ..... 152(14)
Traumas and Orthopedic Diseases – 1418518 .... **152(21)**
Amputation, traumatic – 5451891 .... 152(23)
Ankylosis – 1848522 .... 152(27)
Bursitis – 75184321 .... 152(30)
Contracture, Dupuytren's – 5185421 .... 152(33)
Contracture, joint – 8144855 .... 153(01)
Hallux valgus (Bunion) – 5418521 .... 153(04)
Hemarthrosis – 7184321 .... 153(08)
Pseudarthrosis – 8214231 .... 153(10)
Shock, traumatic – 1454814 .... 153(14)
Sprains (Distortion) – 5148517 .... 153(18)
Trauma, inner organs – 5432188 .... 153(22)

Chapter 23 EAR, NOSE AND THROAT
DISEASES – 1851432 .... 154(07)
Abscess, retropharyngeal – 1454321 .... 154(10)
Adenoids (Tonsil, pharyngeal) – 5189514 .... 154(13)
Aerosinusitis (Sinus barotrauma) – 514854237 .... 154(17)
Angina tonsillaris (Tonsillitis, acute) – 1999999 .... 154(21)
Angiofibroma, nasopharyngeal juvenile – 1111122 .... 154(25)
Atresia, choanal (Synechia, nasal) – 1989142 .... 154(28)
Coryza (Rhinitis, Common cold) – 5189912 .... 154(32)
Deformations, nasal septal – 148543285 .... 155(01)

Ear wax (Cerumen) – 48145814 .... 155(05)
Epistaxis (Nose bleeds) – 65184321 .... 155(08)
Eustachitis – 18554321 .... 155(12)
Foreign objects, ear – 54321545 .... 155(15)
Furuncle, nasal vestibule – 1389145 .... 155(20)
Glottis, edema of – 2314514 .... 155(24)
Hematoma, nasal septum – 5431482 .... 155(28)
Labyrinthitis – 48154219 .... 155(31)
Laryngeal web – 148543283 .... 156(01)
Laryngitis – 4548511 .... 156(05)
Laryngospasm – 485148248 .... 156(07)
Mastoiditis, acute – 514832186 .... 156(11)
Meniere's disease – 514854233 .... 156(15)
Mucocele, frontal sinus (Cyst, mucous) – 5148322 .... 156(19)
Othematoma (Auricular hematoma, Cauliflower ear,
Wrestler's ear) – 4853121 .... 156(23)
Otitis (externa, media, interna) – 55184321 .... 156(28)
Otoantritis (Mastoiditis, chronic) – 1844578 .... 156(32)
Otomycosis – 514832188 .... 157(01)
Otosclerosis (Otospongiosis) – 4814851 .... 157(04)
Ozaena (Rhinitis, atrophic) – 514854241 .... 157(08)
Paralysis, laryngeal – 1854555 .... 157(13)
Pharyngitis – 1858561 .... 157(17)
Pharyngomycosis – 1454511 .... 157(20)
Polyp, nasal – 5519740 .... 157(23)
Rhinitis, vasomotor or allergic (Pollinosis, Hay fever) –
514852351 .... 157(26)
Scleroma (Rhinoscleroma) – 0198514 .... 157(31)
Sepsis, otogenic – 5900001 .... 158(01)
Sinusitis – 1800124 .... 158(06)
Stenosis, laryngeal – 7654321 .... 158(09)
Stridor, congenital (Laryngomalacia) – 4185444 .... 158(14)
Tinnitus – 1488513 .... 158(17)
Tonsillar hypertrophy – 4514548 .... 158(20)
Tonsillitis, acute – 1999999 – see Angina tonsillaris .... 158(24)
Tonsillitis, chronic – 35184321 .... 158(27)
Trauma, ear – 4548515 .... 158(30)
Tuberculosis, laryngeal – 5148541 .... 158(33)
Tumor, larynx – 5148742 .... 159(01)

Chapter 24 EYE DISEASES – 1891014 ...... 160(07)

Amblyopia (Lazy eye) – 1899999 .... 160(10)
Asthenopia (Eye strain) – 9814214..................................... 160(14)
Astigmatism – 1421543 .... 160(17)
Blepharitis – 5142589 .... 160(20)
Cataract – 5189142 .... 160(23)
Chalazion (Eyelid cyst) – 5148582..................................... 160(26)
Chorioiditis – 5182584 .... 160(29)
Conjunctivitis – 5184314.. 160(33)
Dacryocystitis – 45184321 .... 161(01)
Ectopia lentis (Lens displacement) – 25184321 .... 161(04)
Ectropion (Lower eyelid, drooping) – 5142321 .... 161(08)
Endophthalmitis – 514254842... 161(14)
Exophthalmos (Proptosis, Bulging eye) – 5454311............... 161(18)
Eyeball injuries – 518432118 .... 161(22)
Glaucoma (Ocular hypertension) – 5131482........................ 161(25)
Hordeolum (Stye) – 514854249.. 161(31)
Hyperopia (Farsightedness) – 5189988 .... 161(34)
Iritis – 5891231 .... 162(04)
Keratitis – 518432114... 162(07)
Myopia (Nearsightedness) – 548132198 .... 162(09)
Neuritis, optic – 5451589.. 162(13)
Nyctalopia (Night blindness) – 5142842 .... 162(18)
Occlusion, central retinal artery – 514852178....................... 162(21)
Occlusion, central retinal vein – 7777788 .... 162(25)
Ocular burn (Eye burn) – 8881112 .... 162(30)
Ophthalmia, sympathetic – 8185321 .... 162(34)
Optic nerve, atrophy – 5182432.. 163(03)
Panophthalmia – 5141588.. 163(08)
Papilledema (Optic disc edema) – 145432152 .... 163(11)
Photo ophthalmia (Photokeratitis, Snow blindness) –
5841321.. 163(14)
Presbyopia (Farsightedness of the aging) – 1481854 .... 163(18)
Pterygium (Surfer's eye) – 18543212.................................... 163(23)
Ptosis (Upper eyelid, drooping) – 18543121 .... 163(26)
Retinal detachment – 1851760... 163(29)
Retinitis – 5484512 .... 163(33)
Scleritis, Episcleritis – 514854248 .... 164(01)

Strabismus (Tropia, Cross-eyed squint) – 518543254............ 164(06)
Trachoma – 5189523 .... 164(10)
Ulcer, corneal – 548432194 .... 164(13)
Uveitis – 548432198 .... 164(18)
Vernal keratoconjunctivitis (Catarrh, spring) – 514258951.... 164(21)

**Chapter 25 DISEASES OF THE TEETH AND
 ORAL CAVITY – 1488514.........................165(07)**
Abscess, premaxillary – 518231415 .... 165(10)
Alveolitis, dental (Dry socket) – 5848188 .... 165(14)
Bleeding, tooth extraction, after – 8144542.......................... 165(18)
Cheilitis (Chapped lips)– 518431482 .... 165(21)
Cyst, jaw – 514218877 .... 165(24)
Dental calculus (Dental tartar) – 514852182 .... 165(27)
Dental caries (Tooth decay) – 5148584 .... 165(30)
Dental focal infection – 514854814... 165(34)
Gingivitis – 548432123.. 166(04)
Glossalgia (Tongue pain) – 514852181 .... 166(07)
Glossitis (Tongue inflammation) – 1484542............................. 166(10)
Hyperesthesia, teeth – 1484312 .... 166(13)
Hypoplasia, tooth enamel – 74854321.................................... 166(16)
Jaw, fractured – 5182148 .... 166(19)
Leukoplakia – 485148151... 166(22)
Osteomyelitis, jawbone – 5414214....................................... 166(26)
Papillitis, interdental – 5844522 .... 166(30)
Pericoronitis – 5188888 .... 166(33)
Periodontal disease (Paradontosis) – 58145421 .... 167(01)
Periodontitis – 5182821 .... 167(07)
Periodontitis, apical – 3124601.. 167(12)
Phlegmon, maxillofacial region – 5148312 .... 167(17)
Pulpitis – 1468550 .... 167(21)
Stomatitis – 4814854 .... 167(25)
TMJ (temporomandibular joint), ankylosis – 514852179 ...... 167(28)
TMJ (temporomandibular joint), arthritis – 548432174......... 167(33)
TMJ (temporomandibular joint), dislocation (Locked jaw)
– 5484311.. 168(01)
Tooth luxation – 485143277 .... 168(05)
Tooth, fractured (broken) – 814454251 .... 168(09)
Toothache, acute – 5182544 .... 168(12)

Xerostomia (Dry mouth) – 5814514........................ 168(17)

**Chapter 26 UNKNOWN DISEASES AND
CONDITIONS – 1884321 ....169(07)**

**Chapter 27 NORMAL LABORATORY TEST
VALUES – 1489991 ....170(07)**
Blood System – 1481521 .... 171(15)
Urine – 1852155 177
Intestinal Contents - 1485458 180
Saliva – 514821441................................. 181
Gastric Juice – 5148210............................. 181
Bile – 514852188.................................... 184
Biochemistry of the Blood – 514832189 186
Activity Indicators of Neuroendocrine System –
518432121.. 195

Appendix I **199**

Appendix II **207**

Index **218**

Introduction

This book presents the method of improving conditions of health through concentrating on seven, eight and nine digit numbers, which I have received over the course of my practical work. The seven digit number sequences form the foundation of the system. For further specific conditions eight and nine digit numbers are given in the Table of Contents and also throughout the book.

Through immersion in this method of restoring one's health, by concentrating on the number sequences and comparing the various and several number sequences, one can address all aspects of a medical condition.

The method of concentration on the congruent number sequences – after previous and careful diagnosis – provides a possibility to heal people or to improve their situation prophylactically. Furthermore, you can discover the mutual dependencies between several diagnoses. If you take the seven-digit sequence for one disease and another for a different disease, you can receive information from the meaning of the sequences about what connects these diseases with their respective general methods of treatment.

In this manner you can, through an understanding of the situation and its corresponding mental condition, trace a treatment back to the level of a "single impulse." In this case the concentration focuses on a restoration from specific diseases. You can, however, apply this work to any situation requiring a guidance of events within a person's lifetime as well as the revivification of a person after his biological death.

The concentration for the maintenance or the restoration of the body or for the guidance of events can be undertaken by the patient himself or herself. One can, for example, focus upon the number sequence for the appropriate chapter. This is a good method when the disease clearly belongs to this chapter, but the specific diagnosis is missing, for in this man-

01 ner all of the forms of illness belonging to this chapter will
02 be covered.
03   If the diagnosis is known, then you concentrate on the num-
04 bers given for that disease. You can use various methods of
05 concentration. You can take the sequence apart and try to un-
06 derstand how you should order the numbers in order to direct
07 their effect towards best accomplishing a complete restorati-
08 on of health. Develop your own concentration method!
09   The approach described here concerns the general system
10 of guidance of events through concentration on number se-
11 quences. Do the focus by concentrating on the numbers one
12 after another: for example, from the first to the last number, or
13 by selecting individual numbers or sections of the sequence.
14 This gives variation to your focus. The method for your focus
15 can be completely individual according to how you choose
16 to do it.
17   You can undertake your concentration at any time. Just note
18 the number or write it down or use some other method of
19 remembering it.
20   It is important to understand the magnitude of the mental
21 component for the development and removal of diseases and
22 how you can apply this knowledge to man and to a system for
23 the prevention of global catastrophes. The more quickly this
24 knowledge spreads, the faster both individual and collective
25 results will be attained.
26
27
28
29
30
31
32
33
34

CHAPTER 1

CRITICAL CONDITIONS – 1258912

CARDIAC ARREST – 8915678 – is a transition state between life and death. It is not yet death, but it is no longer life. It begins in the moment of discontinuation of the central nervous system, the circulation and the breathing and continues up to the point of irreversible changes in the tissues and primarily in the brain.

CARDIOVASCULAR INSUFFICIENCY, ACUTE (HEART FAILURE, ACUTE) – 1895678 – is the lost ability of the heart to provide the organs and systems with an adequate supply of blood. This is a mismatch between the ability of the heart to pump blood and the oxygen requirements of the tissue. It is characterized by low blood pressure and a decrease in the flow of blood in the tissue.

RESPIRATORY FAILURE, ACUTE – 1257814 – is a pathological condition of the organism in which the normal acid–base balance is not maintained or is achieved through an activity of the compensatory mechanism of the external respiration. This is characterized by the dropping of the pO_2 in the arterial bloodstream (paO_2) to fewer than 50 mm Hg by the intake of atmospheric air; increase of the pCO_2 in the arterial bloodstream ($paCO_2$) to more than 50 mm Hg; disruption of the mechanism and rhythm of the breathing; decrease of the pH value (7.35).

01   **TRAUMATIC SHOCK, SHOCK AND SHOCK–LIKE**
02 **CONDITIONS** – 1895132 – a serious, life-threatening condi-
03 tion caused by trauma and accompanied by disruption in the
04 functioning of the vital organs, in particular circulation and
05 respiration.
06
07
08
09
10
11
12
13
14
15
16
17
18
19
20
21
22
23
24
25
26
27
28
29
30
31
32
33
34

CHAPTER 2

TUMORS – 8214351

CANCER, BLADDER – 89123459 – a malignant tumor that often develops in people who are occupationally exposed to aromatic amines or have a chronic cystitis.

CANCER, BONE – 1234589 – primary malignant bone tumors including osteogenic tumors (paraossal sarcoma, chondrosarcoma, giant cell tumor) and non-osteogenic tumors (Ewing's sarcoma, fibrosarcoma, chondroma, angiosarcoma, and adamantinoma).

CANCER, BREAST – 5432189 – a malignant tumor of the mammary gland. Risk factors include: menopause, age over 50 years, lack of childbearing or the first birth in an age over 30 years, positive family history (breast cancer of the mother, sister or both), fibrocystic breast disease.

CANCER, COLON (COLORECTAL CANCER) – 5821435 – a malignant tumor occurring in the lower, medium or upper part of the rectum that is often diagnosed as adenocarcinoma and more seldom resembles the structure of signet ring cell tumors, undifferentiated or small cell carcinomas.

CANCER, ESOPHAGEAL – 8912567 – a squamous cell cancer that occurs mostly in the middle third of the esophagus.

01   **CANCER, EXTRAHEPATIC BILE DUCT** – 5789154
02 a malignant epithelial tumor forming adenocarcinomas of
03 various differentiation and marked by invasive growth with
04 damage to the ductus choledochus.
05
06   **CANCER, GALLBLADDER** – 8912453 – a malignant epi-
07 thelial tumor, most of which are adenocarcinomas with vari-
08 ous differentiations and the ability to infiltrate the surround-
09 ing tissue and less often forming squamous cell carcinomas
10 (less than 15%).
11
12   **CANCER, KIDNEY** – 56789108 – a renal cell carcinoma
13 arising from the renal cortex and the kidney pelvis (adenocar-
14 cinoma).
15
16   **CANCER, LIPS** – 1567812 – a malignant, squamous cell
17 carcinoma with keratosis, arising from epithelial cells.
18
19   **CANCER, LIVER** – 5891248 – a malignant tumor of the
20 liver most often originating from the liver cell (hepatocellular
21 carcinoma) and occurring less often in the bile duct (cholan-
22 gio carcinoma).
23
24   **LUNG CANCER** – 4541589 – See Chpt 7: *Respiratory*
25 *Diseases, Lung cancer.*
26
27   **CANCER, MAJOR DUODENAL PAPILLA** – 8912345 –
28 a malignant epithelial tumor; in 40% of the cases a primary
29 tumor or an invading tumor originating from the bile ducts,
30 duodenum or pancreas.
31
32   **CANCER, MOUTH AND THROAT** – 1235689 – a squa-
33 mous cell (flat-cell) carcinoma, undifferentiated cancer and
34 lymphoepithelioma, including tumors of the palatine tonsils,
   the roof of the tongue and the retropharynx.

CANCER, OVARIAN – 4851923 – malignant tumor of an ovary. The most common form is the epithelial tumor, including serous, endometrioid and mucinous tumors.

CANCER, PANCREATIC – 8125891 – a malignant tumor localized in the head, body or tail of the pancreas and originating most commonly in the pancreatic duct (ductal adenocarcinoma)

CANCER, PENIS – 8514921 – a well-differentiated squamous cancer that damages the penile shaft.

CANCER, PROSTATE – 4321890 – a malignant tumor occurring as an adenocarcinoma with varying differentiation.

CANCER, SALIVARY GLAND – 9854321 – often occurs as a malignant tumor in the parotid gland and less often in the submandibular and sublingual gland.

CANCER, SKIN – 8148957 – a malignant epithelial tumor occurring on the body surface preceded by the formation of hyperkeratosis. It is age-related and develops due to overexposure to ultraviolet radiation, Bowen's disease, radiation dermatitis, xeroderma pigmentosum, albinism, chronic ulcers, scars, etc.

CANCER, SMALL INTESTINES – 5485143 – a carcinoid tumor or leiomyosarcoma that localizes in the duodenum, the jejunum or the terminal small intestine.

CANCER, STOMACH – 8912534 – a malignant epithelial tumor localized in the upper section (cardia, fundus), middle section (corpus) or lower section (pylorus) of the stomach. It causes non-specific symptoms: nausea, vomiting, eructation,

01 dysphagia, general weakness, weight loss, anemia.
02
03   **CANCER, TESTICULAR** – 5814321 – originates in the
04 germinal epithelium (germ cell tumor) and non-germ cell
05 tumors that are derived from hormone producing cells and
06 the connective tissue (stroma).
07
08   **CANCER, THYROID** – 5814542 – histologically distin-
09 guished as papillary cancer, follicular cancer and more sel-
10 dom as anaplastic and medullary thyroid cancer.
11
12   **CANCER, URETER** – 5891856 – a malignant tumor com-
13 monly occurring in the lower third of the ureter and often
14 similar to bladder cancers.
15
16   **CANCER, VAGINAL AND OF THE EXTERNAL GENI-**
17 **TALS** – 2589121 – a malignant epithelial tumor that stems
18 from precancerous diseases (leukoplakia and kraurosis).
19
20   **CANCER, VULVA** – 5148945 – See Chpt 17: *Obstetrics,*
21 *Gynecological Disorders, Cancer, vulva.*
22
23   **HEMATOSARCOMA AND LYMPHOMA** – 54321451 –
24 see Chpt 10: Blood Diseases: Hemoblastosis outside of bone
25 marrow, Hematosarcoma, and Lymphoma (Lymphocytoma).
26
27   **LEUKEMIA** – 5481347 – see Chpt 10: *Blood Diseases,*
28 *Leukemia.*
29
30   **LYMPHOGRANULOMATOSIS (HODGKIN'S DISEASE)**
31 – 4845714 – see Chpt 10: *Blood Diseases, Lymphogranulo-*
32 *matosis.*
33
34   **LYMPHOMA OF THE SKIN** – 5891243 – a tumorous
disease caused by T and B lymphocytes that become malig-

nant and primarily affect the skin.

MELANOMA – 5674321 – a malignant tumor of melano-cytes found predominantly in skin and less often in conjuncti-vas, choroid coat of the eye, the nasal mucosa, the oral cavity, vagina and rectum.

MESOTHELIOMA – 58912434 – a malignant tumor ori-ginating in the pleura or peritoneum.

NEUROBLASTOMA – 8914567 – a malignant tumor that metastasizes to the skeletal system or liver and originates from the sympathetic nervous system and also the medulla of the adrenal glands.

PLASMOCYTOMA, MULTIPLE MYELOMA, NON-HODGKIN LYMPHOMA – 8432184 – see Chpt 10: *Blood Diseases, Paraproteinemia producing tumors.*

RHABDOMYOSARCOMA IN CHILDREN – 5671254 – a form of sarcoma found in pediatrics and occurring mostly in the soft tissues. There are three histological variations: embryonal, alveolar and pleomorphic. Polymorphic types are mostly found in adults.

SARCOMA, KAPOSI'S – 8214382 – a malignant tumor appearing mostly as skin lesions affecting the trunk or ext-remities and less often the lymph nodes, visceral organs and bones.

SARCOMA, SOFT-TISSUE – 54321891 – a malignant tumor that develops in the connective tissue of the extremi-ties and in the retroperitoneal space and other body regions.

01   **TUMOR, ADRENAL** – 5678123 – neoplasm of the tis-
02 sue of the adrenal gland consisting of altered cells that have
03 become atypical in regard to their growth character and endo-
04 crinal function.
05
06   **TUMOR, BRAIN** – 5451214 – See Chpt 18: *Neurological*
07 *Diseases, Tumor brain.*
08
09   **TUMOR, BRAIN OR SPINAL CORD** – 5431547 – malig-
10 nant tumors in adults and children the most common of which
11 are the glioblastoma and the aggressive astrocytoma.
12
13   **TUMOR, ISLET CELL** – 8951432 – a rare form of pan-
14 creatic tumor, benign or cancerous, derived from the endo-
15 crine part of the pancreas and having a better prognosis than
16 the cancer of the pancreatic duct (Pancreas cancer).
17
18   **TUMOR, NASAL CAVITY AND PARANASAL SINUSES** –
19 8514256 – a squamous cell (flat cell) cancer that is localized
20 in the nasal cavity or in the paranasal sinuses.
21
22   **TUMOR, NASOPHARYNX** – 5678910 – the squamous
23 cell (flat cell) cancer is the most common form of cancer in
24 this area.
25
26   **TUMOR, PARATHYROID** – 1548910 – these are nor-
27 mally benign adenomas but are sometimes cancerous. They
28 are slow growing and metastasize to the nearby lymph nodes,
29 the lung and the liver.
30
31   **TUMOR, PERIPHERAL NERVOUS SYSTEM** –
32 514832182 – See Chpt 18: *Neurological Diseases, Tumor,*
33 *peripheral nervous system.*
34

TUMOR, SPINAL CORD – 51843210 – See Chpt 18: *Neurological Diseases, Tumor, spinal cord.*

TUMOR, UTERUS – 9817453 – malignant tumor of the corpus uteri diagnosed mostly in premenopausal women older than 40 years of age. Obesity, diabetes, hypertension increase the risk of endometrial cancer.

CHAPTER 3

SEPSIS – 58143212

SEPSIS (BLOOD POISONING) –
acute – 8914321; chronic – 8145421 – a condition marked by the progressive spread of bacterial, viral or fungal pathogens throughout the bloodstream.

CHAPTER 4

DISSEMINATED INTRAVASCULAR
COAGULATION (DIC SYNDROME) – 5148142

DISSEMINATED INTRAVASCULAR COAGULATION (DIC SYNDROME, CONSUMPTIVE COAGULOPATHY) – 8123454 – observed in certain diseases, common in sepsis and all terminal conditions; marked by disseminated intravascular coagulation, activation and breakdown of the fibrinolytic system, excess clotting with disruption of microcirculation in organs and tissues, impaired organ perfusion and dysfunction, and excessive thrombolysis leading to hemorrhage.

CHAPTER 5

DISEASES OF THE
CARDIOVASCULAR SYSTEM – 1289435

ANEURYSM, AORTIC – 48543218 – see Chpt 22: *Surgeries, Aneurysm.*

ANEURYSM, CARDIAC – 9187549 – see Chpt 22: *Surgeries.*

ARRHYTHMIA (CARDIAC DYSRHYTHMIA) – 8543210 – created by a disturbance in the heart's electrical system, which affects the heart's ability to pump properly and regularly.

ATHEROSCLEROSIS – 54321898 – the most widely occurring chronic disease, characterized by damage to the elastic arteries (aorta and its branches and arches) and to the muscular-type arteries (heart and brain) with a build-up of fatty materials, primarily of atheromatous plague deposits containing cholesterol on the interior of the arteries.

AUTONOMIC NEUROPATHY (VEGETOVASCULAR DYSTONIA) – 8432910 – a syndrome affecting mostly the cardiovascular system, which refers to a whole range of vascular responses, such as postural (orthostatic) hypotension with tachycardia response, poor R-R variability on ECG and etc. See also: *Neurocirculatory dystonia.*

CARDIAC ASTHMA – 8543214 – sudden shortness of breath due mainly to acute or decompensating chronic left ventricular heart failure with increasing amounts of fluid in the lungs leading to edema.

CARDIALGIA – 8124567 – a feeling of pain in the region of the heart, differing from the pain known as stenocardia and characterized as pricking, burning, pinching, and less often pressing.

CARDIOMYOPATHY (MYOCARDIOPATHY) – 8421432 – primary idiopathic, non-inflammatory damage to the myocardium that is not a result of heart valve defects, intracardiac shunt, arterial or pulmonary hypertension, an ischemic heart disorder or systemic disorders (collagen diseases, amyloidosis, hemochromatosis, etc.).

CARDIOSCLEROSIS – 4891067 – a pathological condition of the heart muscle and its valves caused by growth of connective tissue and scarring (micro- and macro-lesions) in place of functional muscular/valvular tissue.

CIRCULATORY FAILURE – 85432102 – acute or chronic inability of the cardiovascular system to supply the organism and the tissues with enough oxygenated blood to meet their metabolic demands when at rest or under strenuous conditions.

COLLAPSE – 8914320 – a form of acute vascular insufficiency caused by a disturbance in the normal correlation between the capacity of a vessel and the volume of the circulating blood.

CONGENITAL HEART DEFECT – 9995437 – structural abnormalities of the heart and great blood vessels (or both)

01 that occur during intrauterine development affecting the nor-
02 mal flow of blood through the heart and leading to heart fai-
03 lure.
04
05   **COR PULMONALE (PULMONARY HEART DISEASE)** –
06 5432111 – a pathological condition marked by chronic right
07 ventricular hypertrophy and dilatation as a result of high
08 blood pressure in the lungs with a dysfunction in the respira-
09 tory control center.
10
11   **ENDOCARDITIS** – 8145999 – inflammation of the heart
12 valves or the lining of the heart as a result of rheumatic heart
13 disease and less often infections, sepsis, intoxication (uremia)
14 or traumas.
15
16   **HEART BLOCKS** – 9874321 – a problem of the heart's
17 electrical conduction.
18
19   **HEART DEFECT, ACQUIRED** – 8124569 – defects of the
20 heart valves in which they are unable to open fully (stenosis)
21 or close fully (insufficiency) or both (combined defect).
22
23   **HEART FAILURE (CARDIAC FAILURE)** – 8542196 –the
24 inability of the heart to pump enough blood to the rest of the
25 body.
26
27   **HYPERTENSION (HIGH BLOOD PRESSURE)** – 8145432
28 – elevation of the systemic arterial blood pressure.
29
30   **HYPERTENSIVE CRISIS** – 5679102 – extremely high
31 increase in blood pressure in hypertensive diseases, characte-
32 rized by a combination of systemic and regional angiospasms
33 (mainly cerebral).
34

HYPOTENSION (LOW BLOOD PRESSURE) – 8143546 – normally considered as a systolic blood pressure less than 100 mm Hg and diastolic less than 60 mm Hg.

ISCHEMIC HEART DISEASE – IHD (CORONARY HEART DISEASE) – 1454210 – a chronic, pathological process caused by reduced blood supply to the heart muscle. This condition is in most cases due to atherosclerosis of the coronary arteries.

MYOCARDIAL INFARCTION (HEART ATTACK) – 8914325 – a severe heart condition caused by an acute insufficiency in the circulation accompanied by the development of necrosis in the heart muscle. This is the most important clinical form of ischemic heart disease, coronary heart disease.

MYOCARDIODYSTROPHY – 8432110 – non-inflammatory pathology of the cardiac muscle as a result of metabolic disturbances caused by extracardiac factors.

MYOCARDITIS – 85432104 – inflammation of the heart muscle.

NEUROCIRCULATORY DYSTONIA – 5432150 – a variation of Da Costa syndrome (Vegetative dystonia) caused by changes in vascular tone and reactivity due to dystonia (dysfunction) of vasomotor centers (both central and peripheral) of congenital or acquired character. See also: Vegetovascular dystonia.

OCCLUSION OF MAJOR ARTERIES – 81543213 – see Chpt 22: *Surgeries, Occlusion of major arteries.*

PERICARDITIS – 9996127 – acute or chronic inflammation of the pericardial sac.

PULMONARY EDEMA (LUNG EDEMA) – 54321112 – acute shortness of breath (dyspnea) mostly caused by an accumulation of serous fluid in lung tissue and alveoli due to left ventricular heart failure.

RHEUMATIC HEART DISEASE (RHEUMATIC FEVER) – 5481543 – see Chpt 6: *Rheumatic Diseases: Rheumatic heart disease.*

STENOCARDIA (ANGINA PECTORIS) – 8145999 – sudden severe chest pain caused by acute lack of oxygen (ischemia) in the heart muscle; a clinical form of ischemic heart disease and a cause of coronary artery disease.

SYSTEMIC VASCULITIS – 1894238 – see Chpt 6: *Rheumatic Diseases, Systemic vasculitis.*

THROMBOPHLEBITIS – 1454580 – see Chpt 22: *Surgeries: Phlebothrombosis.*

VARICOSIS – 4831388 – see Chpt 22: *Surgeries, Varicosis.*

VASCULAR CRISIS – 8543218 – an acute disturbance of the systemic hemodynamic or the local blood flow caused by a dysfunction of the vascular tone through hypertonia or hypotonia of the arteries, hypotonia of the veins, or a dysfunction of arterial or venous anastomosis in a tissue.

VASCULAR INSUFFICIENCY – 8668888 – a disturbance in the normal correlation between the capacity of a vessel and the volume of the circulating blood due to insufficient vessel tone or a decreased volume of circulating blood or both.

CHAPTER 6

RHEUMATIC DISEASES – 8148888

JOINTS DISEASES – 5421891

ARTHRITIS PSORIATICA – 0145421 – inflammation of the joints with particular features like diffuse swelling of the entire toe in patients with Psoriasis.

ARTHRITIS, DEGENERATIVE (OSTEOARTHRITIS, OSTEOARTHROSIS, ARTHROSIS DEFORMANS, DEGE-NERATIVE JOINT DISEASE) – 8145812 – a non-inflammatory joint disease marked by progressive cartilage degeneration.

ARTHRITIS, REACTIVE – (REITER'S SYNDROME) – 4848111 – a disease marked by the classic triad of arthritis, urethritis and conjunctivitis, sometimes also a peculiar dermatitis.

ARTHRITIS, RHEUMATOID – 8914201 – a systemic, chronic inflammation disorder of the connective tissues, mainly causing chronic progressive inflammation of the joints.

CONNECTIVE TISSUE DISEASE, MIXED (SHARP'S SYNDROME) – 1484019 – overlapping clinical features of skleroderma, systemic lupus erythematosus and rheumatoid arthritis. See also *Connective tissue disease, diffuse.*

CONNECTIVE TISSUE DISEASES, DIFFUSE – 5485812 – a group of disorders marked by systemic immunocomplex inflammation, autoimmune reactions and formation of fibrosis. See also *Connective tissue disease, mixed.*

CRYSTAL DEPOSITION DISEASE SYNDROME – 0014235 – a group of joint diseases caused by deposits of microcrystals (e.g. gout and pseudogout).

DERMATOMYOSITIS (POLYMYOSITIS) – 5481234 – a systemic connective tissue disease affecting muscles or groups of muscles and skin.

GIANT-CELL ARTERITIS (CRANIAL ARTERITIS, TEMPORAL ARTERITIS, HORTON'S DISEASE) – 9998102 – a systemic vasculitis affecting the large arteries of the head and leading to granulomatous inflammation with giant cells in the medial layers of the arteries.

GOODPASTURE'S SYNDROME (GLOMERULONEPHRITIS, HEMORRHAGIC PNEUMONIA) – 8491454 – a systemic autoimmune disorder mainly affecting the lungs and kidneys that is marked by pulmonary hemorrhage and glomerulonephritis.

HEMORRHAGIC VASCULITIS (ALLERGIC VASCULITIS, PURPURA HENOCH-SCHOENLEIN) – 8491234 – systemic damage to the capillaries, arterioles, and venules mainly in the skin, joints, abdomen and kidneys.

INFECTIOUS ARTHRITIS – 8111110 – infection of one or more joints caused by bacteria, viruses or fungi.

LUPUS ERYTHEMATOSUS – 8543148 – a chronic, systemic autoimmune disease of the connective tissue and the blood vessels.

PERIARTHRITIS – 4548145 – inflammation of the tissues around a joint (tendon, bursa, capsule) without evidence of arthritis.

PODAGRA (GOUT) – 8543215 – disorder of the purine metabolism characterized by the deposition of uric acid in the organism.

POLYARTERITIS NODOSA (PERIARTERITIS NODOSA, KUSSMAUL DISEASE) – 54321894 – a serious systemic blood vessel disease with inflammation of the small arteries and nodular thickening of the tunica adventitia.

RHEUMATIC HEART DISEASE (RHEUMATIC FEVER) – 5481543 – a systemic infectious disease of the connective tissue mostly affecting the heart. See also Chpt 5: *Endocarditis* – 8145999.

RHEUMATISM, SOFT TISSUE NEAR JOINT – 1489123 – diseases of the tendons (Tendinitis, Tendovaginitis), ligaments, the site of attachment of these structures to the bone (Enthesopathy), bursae (Bursitis), aponeuroses and fasciae of inflammatory or degenerative character. These conditions are not caused by trauma, injuries, infections or tumors.

SJOEGREN'S SYNDROME (SICCA SYNDROME, MIKULICZ DISEASE) – 4891456 – a rheumatoid autoimmune disease affecting the moisture producing and sebaceous glands with decreased production of tears and saliva with symptoms like keratoconjunctivitis, parotitis, and pancreatic insufficiency.

SKLERODERMA, SYSTEMIC – 1110006 – a systemic autoimmune disease of the connective tissues with thickening of the skin and the formation of scar tissue (progressive fibrosis).

SPONDYLITIS ANKYLOPOETICA (BECHTEREW'S DISEASE, MARIE-STRUEMPELL DISEASE) – 4891201 – a chronic, systemic inflammatory disease affecting the joints of the spine with progressive impaired mobility.

SYSTEMIC VASCULITIS (SV) – 1894238 – refers to a number of conditions characterized by systemic inflammations of small vessels (both arteries and veins can be affected).

TAKAYASU'S ARTERITIS – 8945432 – a systemic disease marked by inflammation of the aorta and its major branches with development of partial or complete obstruction of the affected blood vessel.

TENDOVAGINITIS – 1489154 – inflammation of a tendon and its sheath.

THROMBANGIITIS OBLITERANS (BUERGER'S DISEASE) – 8945482 – a systemic inflammatory disease of the artery (Thromboarteriitis) or vein (Thrombophlebitis) leading to obstruction of the blood vessels involved.

WEGENER'S GRANULOMATOSIS – 8943568 – a granulomatous inflammation of the respiratory system, the lungs and the kidneys.

CHAPTER 7

RESPIRATORY DISEASES – 5823214

ANTHRACOSIS – 5843214 – a severe form of coal worker's pneumoconiosis caused by the long-term exposure to coal dust.

ASBESTOSIS – 4814321 – a form of pneumoconiosis and silicosis caused by inhalation of asbestos fibers.

ASPERGILLOSIS – 481543271 – caused by fungi of the genus Aspergillus. The most common form affects the respiratory organs, e.g. pulmonary aspergillosis, pneumomycosis, otomycosis, keratomycosis.

ASTHMA, BRONCHIAL – 8943548 – an allergic disorder with short attacks of dyspnea due to spastic contractions of the bronchioles (bronchospasm).

BRONCHIOLITIS (BRONCHIOLES, ACUTE INFLAM-MATION OF) – 89143215 – acute inflammation of the small air passages of the lung, considered to be a severe form of acute bronchitis.

BRONCHITIS, ACUTE – 4812567 – an acute, diffuse inflammation of the tracheobronchial tree.

BRONCHITIS, CHRONIC – 4218910 – a diffuse, progressive inflammation of the bronchial airways with productive

01 cough and no local, generalized damage of the lung tissue.
02
03   **COAL WORKER'S PNEUMOCONIOSIS (CARBOCONI-**
04 **OSIS, BLACK LUNG DISEASE)** – 8148545 – caused by inha-
05 lation of carbon dust from coal, graphite or soot and marked
06 by the development of nodular lesions and fibrosis.
07
08   **EMPHYSEMA, LUNG** – 54321892 – a frequently chronic
09 condition marked by pathologic enlargement of the airspaces
10 distal to the terminal bronchiole and accompanied by the
11 destruction of their walls.
12
13   **LUNG FIBROSIS (PNEUMOSCLEROSIS)** – 9871234 – a
14 chronic condition of the lung and complication after various
15 lung diseases (pneumonia, chronic bronchitis, tuberculosis,
16 syphilis).
17
18   **METALLOCONIOSIS** – 4845584 – caused by inhalation
19 of dust containing metals and metal alloys (Beryllisosis –
20 beryllium dust exposure; Siderosis – exposure to dust with
21 iron salts; Aluminosis – aluminum dust exposure; Baritosis
22 – barium dust exposure).
23
24   **PLEURITIS (PLEURISY)** – 4854444 – inflammation of
25 the lining of the lungs with fibrinous exudation upon its sur-
26 face or into its cavity.
27
28   **PNEUMOCONIOSIS** – 8423457 – an occupational lung
29 disease due to chronic inhalation of mineral or metal dust par-
30 ticles causing changes to the lung tissue and development of
31 diffuse interstitial fibrosis.
32
33   **PNEUMOCONIOSIS OF ORGANIC DUST** – 4548912 – a
34 more benign form of pneumoconiosis caused by inhalation of
    organic dust (cotton, grain, cork, reed, etc.).

PNEUMONIA – 4814489 – a group of inflammatory diseases of the lung affecting the lung parenchyma (alveoli). There are two anatomical forms: lobar pneumonia and bronchopneumonia with multiple lesions that are focally distributed and affect one or more lobules.

PNEUMONITIS, ACUTE INTERSTITIAL (HAMMAN–RICH SYNDROME) – 4814578 – a rapidly progressive, diffuse interstitial lung fibrosis occurring in patients without preexisting lung disease; prognosis is usually poor.

PULMONARY CANCER (LUNG CANCER) – 4541589 – 98% of primary lung cancers originate from the bronchial walls.

PULMONARY CANDIDIASIS (CANDIDIASIS OF THE LUNG) – 4891444 – See also Chpt 8: *Digestive System, Candidiasis* – marked by the appearance of fine pneumonic infiltrates with central necrosis and mucosal exudate in the alveoli.

PULMONARY INFARCTION (LUNG INFARCTION) – 89143211 – tissue death due to local lack of oxygen mostly in peripheral lung areas through obstruction or vasoconstriction.

SARCOIDOSIS – 4589123 – a systemic disease marked by the formation of granulomas consisting of epithelioid cells, multinucleated giant cells, Langhans giant cells and foreign-body giant cells.

SILICATOSIS – 2224698 – develops through the chronic inhalation of dust containing silicon dioxide and also other minerals such as magnesium, calcium, iron, and aluminum.

SILICOSIS (POTTER'S ROT) – 4818912 – the most common and severe form of pneumoconiosis resulting from chronic (occupational) inhalation of mineral dust particles containing silicon dioxide.

TALCOSIS – 4845145 – a relatively benign form of silicatosis caused by inhalation of dust containing talc and silicates.

TUBERCULOSIS, PULMONARY – 8941234 – a serious infectious disease characterized by specific inflammatory infiltration and formation of tubercles; affects the whole organism.

CHAPTER 8

DISEASES OF THE DIGESTIVE SYSTEM – 5321482

ACHALASIA OF CARDIA (CARDIOSPASM, HIATO-SPASM, MEGAESOPHAGUS, IDIOPATHIC DILATION OF ESOPHAGUS) – 4895132 – a condition marked by dysphagia, regurgitation of food, and heartburn and caused by degeneration of the nerve cells that normally signal the brain to relax the esophageal sphincter. This prevents the normal act of swallowing. If the esophageal sphincter remains contracted, normal peristalsis is interrupted and food cannot enter the stomach.

ACHYLIA GASTRICA – 8432157 – the absence of gastric juices without the presence of any organic damage to the secretion producing mechanisms of the stomach.

AMOEBIASIS –1289145 – see Chpt 14: *Infectious Diseases.*

AMYLOIDOSIS – 5432185 – metabolic disorder caused by abnormal deposition of amyloid proteins in organs and tissues (esp. liver, spleen, and kidneys).

ATONIA OF THE ESOPHAGUS AND THE STOMACH – 8123457 – see *Dyskinesia of the digestive tract.*

BERIBERI – 3489112 – a lack of Vitamin B1 (thiamine), endemic in Asia (see also Chpt 15:*Vitamin Deficiency Diseases).*

BRONZE DIABETES – 5454589 – see Hemochromatosis.

CANDIDIASIS (THRUSH, YEAST INFECTION) – 54842148 – a group of diseases, which are caused by a fungal infection of any of the Candida (yeast) species.

CARCINOID SYNDROME – 4848145 – a rare and slow-growing, hormone producing tumor originating in the cells of the neuroendocrine system

CARDIOSPASM – 4895132 – see *Achalasia of cardia.*

CHOLECYSTITIS, ACUTE – 4154382 – see Chpt 22: *Surgical Diseases.*

CHOLECYSTITIS, CHRONIC – 5481245 – chronic inflammation of the gallbladder.

CHOLECYSTOLITHIASIS – 0148012 – see Chpt 22: *Surgical Diseases.*

CIRRHOSIS OF THE LIVER – 4812345 – a chronic, advanced liver disease marked by evident damage of the lobular structures, hyperplasia of the splenic and hepatic reticulo-endothelial system, and liver dysfunction.

CIRRHOSIS, PIGMENT – 5454589 – see Hemochromatosis.

COLITIS – 8454321 – inflammation of the large intestine.

COLITIS, ACUTE – 5432145 – widespread condition often combined with an acute inflammation of the mucous membranes of the small intestine (acute enterocolitis) and sometimes also with an inflammation of the stomach.

COLITIS, CHRONIC – 5481238 – common disorder of the digestive system often combined with inflammatory conditions of the small intestine (enterocolitis).

CONSTIPATION – 5484548 – decreased frequency of bowel elimination, multiple causes.

DIARRHEA – 5843218 – three or more liquid or loose bowel movements a day accompanied by rapid passage of food, due to increased peristalsis, failure of fluid resorption in the colon, and secretion of inflammatory exudate or transudate.

DIARRHEA, FUNCTIONAL – 81234574 – see *Dyskinesia of the digestive tract.*

DUODENAL STASIS – 8123457 – see *Dyskinesia of the digestive tract.*

DUODENITIS – 5432114 – inflammation of the duodenum.

DUODENITIS, ACUTE – 481543288 – often combined with acute inflammation of the stomach and intestines and diagnosed as acute gastroenteritis or gastroenterocolitis (catarrhal, ulcerous, erosive, or phlegmonous).

DUODENITIS, CHRONIC – 8432154 – often caused by poor diet with consumption of irritating foods and beverages or alcoholism.

DYSBIOSIS, INTESTINAL (DYSBACTERIOSIS, INTESTINAL) – 5432101 – a syndrome marked by a disturbed balance of the bacterial flora in the gut.

DYSKINESIA OF THE DIGESTIVE TRACT (DYSPEP-SIA; GASTROPTOSIS; DIARRHEA, FUNCTIONAL) – 81234574 – a functional disorder marked by disturbed tonus and peristalsis of the digestive organs consisting of smooth muscle (esophagus, stomach, biliary tract, intestines).

DYSKINESIA, BILIARY – 58432144 – functional disorder of the bile ducts, especially an altered tonus of the sphincter of Oddi.

DYSKINESIA, INTESTINES – 54321893 – includes a broad spectrum of nervous conditions of the intestines with disturbance of the bowel reflexes (irritable bowel syndrome, colon neurosis, spastic colon) and reflex disturbances in other portions of the digestive system (ulcer, cholecystitis, cholecystolithiasis, appendicitis, anal fissure) and in other organs and systems (urolithiasis, adnexitis, etc.).

DYSPEPSIA (INDIGESTION) – 1112223 – can be caused by a variety of conditions such as disturbed digestion, upset stomach, functional disorders of the stomach, insufficient or disturbed production of digestive enzymes or bad diet.

DYSPEPSIA, FUNCTIONAL (HYPERACIDITY, STOMACH) – 5484214 – functional disorders of the stomach with unknown cause marked by excessive excretion of hydrochloric acid.

ENTERITIS – 8431287 – inflammation of the small intestine.

ENTERITIS, CHRONIC – 5432140 – the chronic form of enteritis sometimes involves the jejunum (jejunitis) or the ileum (ileitis).

ENTEROCOLITIS – 8454321 – see *Colitis; Enteritis.*

ENTEROPATHY, DISACCHARIDASE DEFICIENCY – 4845432 – this deficiency disables digestion of lactose (milk sugar), sucrose (cane and beet sugar) and maltose (malt sugar).

ENTEROPATHY, EXUDATIVE – 48123454 – a rare disease with abnormal loss of protein into the gastrointestinal tract, enlarged lymph vessels and diarrhea.

ENTEROPATHY, GLUTEN-INDUCED (CELIAC SPRUE; NONTROPICAL SPRUE; STEATORRHEA, IDIOPATHIC) – 4891483 – an inherited disease of the small intestine characterized by damage to the mucosal lining known as villous atrophy, which leads to malabsorption due to a reaction to gluten.

ENTEROPATHY, OF THE INTESTINES – 8432150 – a general term for non-inflammatory, chronic intestinal conditions; probable causes are enzyme dysfunctions or congenital anomalies of the intestinal wall.

ESOPHAGISM – 5481248 – contraction of the esophagus, differentiated into primary esophagism as a result of disturbances in cortical regulation of the functions of the esophagus and secondary esophagism, which results from Esophagitis ulcers and cholecystolithiasis (gallstones).

ESOPHAGITIS – 54321489 – inflammation of the esophagus; differentiated into acute, subacute and chronic esophagitis.

ESOPHAGOSPASM – 8123457 – see *Dyskinesia of the digestive tract and Esophagus spasm.*

01   **ESOPHAGUS, PEPTIC ULCER** – 8432182 – caused when
02 the lining of the lower esophagus is corroded by the acidic
03 digestive juices secreted by the stomach cells.
04
05   **FOOD ALLERGY** – 2841482 – an allergic response of
06 the digestive organs towards certain foods caused by medica-
07 tions, bacteria, or other substances.
08
09   **GASTRITIS** – 5485674 – inflammation of the lining of
10 the stomach (often also affecting deeper layers of the gastric
11 mucosa).
12
13   **GASTRITIS, ACUTE** – 4567891 – a condition resulting
14 from multiple causes: bacterial, chemicals, various medica-
15 tions, physical stress, thermic irritants, which lead to inflam-
16 mation of and dystrophic-necrobiotic damage to the lining of
17 the stomach.
18
19   **GASTRITIS, CHRONIC** – 5489120 – chronic inflamma-
20 tion of the lining of the stomach (sometimes also affecting
21 deeper layers of the stomach walls).
22
23   **GASTROCARDIAL SYNDROME (ROEMHELD SYN-**
24 **DROME)** – 5458914 – heart symptoms (pain and pressure in
25 the heart region, disturbance to the heart rhythm) due to irrita-
26 tion of the stomach lining arising after eating or with an ulcer
27 or cancer in the cardiac region of the stomach.
28
29   **GASTROENTERITIS** – 5485674 – see *Gastritis, Enteritis.*
30
31   **GASTROENTEROCOLITIS** – 5485674 – see *Gastritis,*
32 *Enteritis.*
33
34   **GASTROINTESTINAL TUBERCULOSIS** – 8143215 –
a rare condition occurring mostly in people with forms of

advanced pulmonary tuberculosis.

GASTROPARESIS (GASTRIC ATONY, ACUTE) – 5485671 – Paralysis of the stomach muscle due to damage to the vagus nerve or triggered by other acute conditions of the abdomen.

GASTROPTOSIS – 81234574 – see *Dyskinesia of the digestive tract.*

HEMOCHROMATOSIS (PIGMENT CIRRHOSIS, BRONZE DIABETES, IRON OVERLOAD DISEASE, SIDEROPHILIA, TROISIER-HANOT-CHAUFFARD SYNDROME) – 5454589 – an inherited disease with accelerated iron absorption resulting in iron overload in the blood and iron deposition in inner organs and tissues.

HEPATIC INSUFFICIENCY (LIVER FAILURE) – 8143214 – deterioration of liver functions as result of acute and chronic damage to the liver tissue.

HEPATITIS – 5814243 – inflammation of the liver.

HEPATITIS, ACUTE – 58432141 – acute form of liver inflammation caused virally (hepatitis A or B, enterovirus) or non-virally (salmonella, leptospira and other pathogens). See also Chpt 14: *Infectious Diseases, Hepatitis, viral A and B* – 5412514.

HEPATITIS, CHRONIC – 5123891 – a chronic (lasting more than 6 months) liver disease with inflammatory dystrophic character and mild to moderate fibrosis, the lobular structure remaining mostly intact.

HEPATOLENTICULAR DEGENERATION (WILSON-KONOWALOW DISEASE) – 5438912 – a disorder marked by dysfunction of the copper metabolism damaging the liver and nervous system (liver cirrhosis, brain degeneration).

HEPATOSIS – 9876512 – a liver disease with predominance of degeneration (dystrophy). One differentiates between acute and chronic hepatosis, the latter is broken down into hepatic steatosis (fatty liver) and cholestatic hepatosis.

HEPATOSIS, ACUTE (LIVER DAMAGE, TOXIC) – 1234576 – fatty degeneration develops into yellow degeneration resulting in massive hepatic necrosis.

HEPATOSIS, CHOLESTATIC (CHOLESTASIS) – 5421548 – characterized by cholestasis and deposition of bile in the hepatocytes along with mainly albuminous degeneration.

HEPATOSIS, CHRONIC (FATTY LIVER, HEPATIC STE-ATOSIS) – 5143214 – marked by chronic fatty dystrophy of the hepatocytes.

HEPATOSPLENOMEGALIC LIPOIDOSIS – 4851888 – see *Hyperlipidemia.*

HEPATOSPLENOMEGALY SYNDROME (HEPATOLIE-NALIC SYNDROME) – 8451485 – enlargement of the liver and spleen of various origins.

HYPERBILIRUBINEMIA, BENIGN – 84514851 – a group of diseases and syndromes marked by yellow discoloration of the skin and mucous membranes, hyperbilirubinemia with normal liver values, and by the lack of morphological changes in the liver. Congenital hyperbilirubinemia and

01 the posthepatitic syndrome also belong to this group.

03   **HYPERBILIRUBINEMIA, CONGENITAL** – 8432180 –
04 a group of inherited diseases with excess of bilirubin in the
05 blood, non-hemolytic jaundice.

07   **HYPERBILIRUBINEMIA, POSTHEPATIC (OBSTRUC-**
08 **TIVE JAUNDICE)** – 8214321 – a jaundice due to gallstones
09 or pancreatic cancer with elevated levels of bilirubin in the
10 blood.

12   **HYPERLIPIDEMIA, IDIOPATHIC (HYPERLIPRO-**
13 **TEINEMIA, HEPATOSPLENOMEGALIC LIPOIDOSIS)** –
14 4851888 – an inherited abnormal lipid metabolism resulting
15 in increased blood fats.

17   **HYPOVITAMINOSIS** – 5154231 – see Chpt 15: *Vitamin*
18 *Deficiency Diseases.*

20   **ILEITIS** – 8431287 – see *Enteritis.*

22   **ILEOCECAL VALVE INFLAMMATION (BAUHINITIS)** –
23 58432148 – inflammation of the Ileocecal valve.

25   **INDIGESTION** – 9988771 – a complexity of symptoms
26 marked by disturbances of the digestive tract (see also: *Dys-*
27 *pepsia*).

29   **INSUFFICIENCY OF THE CARDIAC SPHINCTER** –
30 8545142 – hiatal hernia with resulting insufficiency of the
31 cardia sphincter usually caused by and side effect of surgery
32 or systemic sclerodermia.

34   **JAUNDICE (ICTERUS)** – 5432148 – yellowish pigmenta-
tion of the skin and mucous membranes caused by accumu-

lation of bilirubin in blood and tissues. There are three differentiations: prehepatic, hepatic and posthepatic (obstructive) jaundice.

JAUNDICE, FUNCTIONAL – 84514851 – see *Hyperbilirubinemia, functional.*

JEJUNITIS – 8431287 – see *Enteritis.*

LIPODYSTROPHY, INTESTINAL (WHIPPLE'S DISEASE) – 4814548 – systemic disease with damage mostly to the small intestine resulting in malabsorption (poor fat absorption).

LIVER DYSTROPHY – 9876512 – see *Hepatosis.*

LYMPHANGIECTASIA OF THE COLON – 5214321 – see also *Enteropathy of the colon.*

MALABSORPTION – 48543215 – a complexity of symptoms caused by abnormal absorption of nutrients across the gastrointestinal tract.

PANCREATITIS, ACUTE – 4881431 – see Chpt 22: *Surgical Diseases.*

PANCREATITIS, CHRONIC – 5891432 – chronic inflammation of the pancreas.

PEPTIC ULCER DISEASE OF THE STOMACH AND DUODENUM – 8125432 – a chronic, recurrent disease in which an ulcer forms in the stomach and duodenum due to disturbances of the neural and humoral secretory mechanisms.

PNEUMATOSIS, GASTRIC – 54321455 – air within the stomach wall.

PORTAL HYPERTENSION – 8143218 – a group of symptoms marked by high blood pressure of the portal vein, enlarged portocarval anastomoses, ascites and splenomegaly.

POST-HEPATITIS SYNDROME – 4812819 – a complex of symptoms characterized by a slight hyperbilirubinemia with increased amounts of indirect (unconjugated) bilirubin in the blood; a condition after acute hepatitis with no pathological changes in the liver tissue.

SCURVY – 5432190 – see also Chpt 15: *Diseases from a Lack of Vitamins: Vitamin C deficiency* – 4141255.

SPASM, INTESTINAL (COLIC, INTESTINAL) – 8123457 – see *Dyskinesia of the digestive tract.*

SPRUE, NONTROPICAL – 8432150 – see *Enteropathy, of the intestines.*

SPRUE, TROPICAL (DIARRHEA, TROPICAL) – 5481215 – a chronic and severe disease marked by abnormal flattening of the villi and inflamed lining of the small intestine together with persistent diarrhea, glossitis, and normochromic anemia.

STARVATION EDEMA (HUNGER EDEMA, FAMINE DROPSY, ALIMENTARY DYSTROPHY) – 5456784 – famine dropsy as a result of malnutrition (esp. lack of whole protein) and marked by emaciation, disturbed metabolism and dystrophy of tissues and organs.

01   **STOMACH PHLEGMON** – 4567891 – see *Gastritis,*
02 *acute.*
03
04   **STOMACH ULCERS, SYMPTOMATIC** – 9671428 – acute
05 or chronic lesions of the mucous membranes of the stomach;
06 differs from peptic ulcer disease in its etiology and pathology.
07
08   **SUPERIOR MESENTERIC ARTERY (SMA) SYNDROME**
09 – 5891234 – a symptom complex caused by compression of
10 the mesenteric artery in the lower horizontal portion of the
11 duodenum.
12
13   **ULCER OF THE SMALL INTESTINE, SIMPLE NONS-**
14 **PECIFIC** – 48481452 – marked by the appearance of single
15 or multiple ulcerations (nonspecific, idiopathic, peptic, tro-
16 phic, round, etc.), primarily in the ileum, which are similar in
17 their morphology to ulcers of the stomach and the duodenum.
18
19   **WHIPPLE'S DISEASE** – 4814548 – see *Lipodystrophy,*
20 *intestinal.*
21
22   **ZINGA** – 54321481 – see Chpt 15: *Diseases from a Lack*
23 *of Vitamins: Vitamin C deficiency.*
24
25
26
27
28
29
30
31
32
33
34

CHAPTER 9

DISEASES OF THE KIDNEYS AND
URINARY TRACT – 8941254

AMYLOIDOSIS – 4512345 – in most cases a systemic disease marked by the deposition of amyloid proteins in organs and tissues resulting in the dysfunction of multiple organs.

CYSTITIS – 48543211 – infection of the bladder caused by invasion of pathogenic bacteria.

GLOMERULONEPHRITIS (DIFFUSE PROLIFERATIVE GN) – 4812351 – an autoimmune disorder that damages the glomeruli.

GLOMERULONEPHRITIS, ACUTE – 4285614.

HYDRONEPHROSIS – 5432154 – distension of the kidney pelvis from urine, usually caused by backward pressure when the flow of urine is obstructed; complications: structural damage to kidney with decreased kidney function.

KIDNEY DISEASE, CHRONIC (KIDNEY FAILURE, CHRONIC) – 5488821.

NEPHROLITHIASIS (KIDNEY STONES) – 5432143 – a condition in which calculi (stones) are formed in the kidneys or urinary tract.

POLYCYSTIC KIDNEY DISEASE (PKD) – 5421451 – a congenital disorder in which multiple cysts grow in the kidneys damaging the healthy kidney tissue in the process.

PROSTRATE ADENOMA – 51432144 – See Chpt 22: *Surgical Diseases, Prostrate adenoma.*

PYELITIS – 5432110 – inflammation of the renal pelvis

PYELONEPHRITIS – 58143213 – a nonspecific infectious disease affecting the kidney tissue, the pelvis, the interstitium and the calyx.

RENAL COLIC – 4321054 – a syndrome marked by acute pain in the lumbar area and observed in a number of diseases of the kidney.

RENAL ECLAMPSIA – 8149141 – see also Glomerulonephritis, acute and Chpt 17: *Obstetrics, Toxemia, in pregnancy (Pre-eclampsia).*

RENAL FAILURE (KIDNEY FAILURE) – 4321843 – a syndrome caused by severe dysfunction of the kidney leading to disruption of the homeostasis and marked by elevated levels of urea nitrogen in the blood, metabolic acidosis, and dysfunction of the acid-base balance (metabolic acidosis).

RENAL FAILURE, ACUTE (KIDNEY FAILURE, ACUTE) – 8218882.

RENAL INSUFFICIENCY – 4321843 – see *Renal failure.*

RENAL TUBERCULOSIS (TUBERCULOSIS OF THE KIDNEY) – 5814543 – an infectious disease caused by bacteria (Mycobacterium tuberculosis) that damages the kidneys.

UREMIA, ACUTE – 5421822 – see also *Renal failure, acute.*

UREMIA, CHRONIC – 8914381 – see also *Kidney disease, chronic.*

URETHRITIS – 1387549 – inflammation of the urethra often due to gonorrhea and sometimes to prostatitis.

URINARY SYSTEM, ANOMALIES – 1234571 – these conditions are mostly congenital defects.

CHAPTER 10

BLOOD DISEASES – 1843214

AGRANULOCYTOSIS – 4856742 – severe lack or abnormal reduction of white blood cells (less than 1000 in 1 µL blood) or granulocytes (less than 750 in 1 µL of blood).

ANEMIA – 48543212 – decrease in hemoglobin in a given unit amount of blood (except for acute blood loss).

ANEMIA OF LEAD POISONING – 1237819 – caused by the interference of lead with heme and other porphyrin synthesis.

ANEMIA, APLASTIC (HYPOPLASTIC) – 5481541 – a group of blood diseases characterized by the absence of the production of all formed elements of the blood leading to the depression of all blood cells in the bone marrow and peripheral blood.

ANEMIA, AUTOIMMUNE HEMOLYTIC – 5814311 – malfunction of the immune system where the autoantibodies attack the body's own red blood cells.

ANEMIA, CONGENITAL; TOGETHER WITH A DISRUPTION OF THE SYNTHESIS OF PORPHYRINE – 4581254 – (sideroblastic anemia) characterized by a lack of hemoglobin in the red blood cells, an increased serum iron level, iron deposits (hemosiderin) with hemosiderosis in the inner organs.

ANEMIA, HEMOLYTIC – 5484813 – the abnormal break-down of red blood cells.

ANEMIA, MEGALOBLASTIC – 5481254 – a group of anemias, which are in general marked by abnormally large red blood cells (megaloblasts) in bone marrow and multi-segmented neutrophils in the peripheral blood.

ANEMIA, POSTHEMORRHAGIC ACUTE (BLOOD LOSS, ACUTE) – 9481232 – acute anemia resulting from excessive bleeding.

ANEMIA, SICKLE-CELL – 7891017 – a large group of diseases determined by an abnormality of the globin genes in the hemoglobin. Hemoglobinopathy is the most common form of sickle-cell anemia.

CHEMOTHERAPY, SIDE EFFECTS OF – 4812813 – includes numerous symptoms as a side effect of chemothe-rapy with destruction mainly of the dividing cells primarily affecting the bone marrow and the cells of the digestive tract. Often accompanied by toxic damage to the liver.

FAVISM – 54321457 – the development of an acute hemo-lytic syndrome in some people with glucose-6-phosphate dehydrogenase (G6PDH) after eating fava beans or inhaling the pollen of this plant.

GAUCHER'S DISEASE – (CEREBROSIDE LIPOIDO-SIS) – 5145432 – a rare hereditary disorder of the cerebroside metabolism resulting in the accumulation of fatty substance in the so-called macrophages (Gaucher's cells) and in certain organs, in particular the spleen, liver and bone marrow.

HEMOBLASTOSIS OUTSIDE OF BONE MARROW, HEMATOSARCOMA, AND LYMPHOMA (LYMPHOCYTOMA) – 54321451 – malignant blood disorders that in the beginning stages do not attack the bone marrow. They can develop from blast cells (hemosarcoma) and mature lymphocytes (lymphosarcoma or lymphocytes).

HEMORRHAGIC DIATHESIS – 5148543 – an unusual tendency to bleeding.

HEMORRHAGIC DIATHESIS, CAUSED BY A PATHOLOGY OF THE BLOOD VESSELS – 54815438 – Osler-Weber-Rendu disease (hereditary hemorrhagic telangiectasia).

HYPOPROTHROMBINEMIA – 5481542 – a hemorrhagic disorder characterized by an acquired or congenital deficit of the prothrombin complex.

LEUKEMIA – 5481347 – malignant disease of the blood building system with increase of abnormal (white) blood cells affecting the bone marrow.

LEUKEMOID REACTIONS – 5814321 – a blood picture resembling CGL (chronic granulocytic leukemia) or other tumors of the blood system, but possibly appearing with some infections (mononucleosis, whooping cough, tuberculosis) or in non-neoplastic dyscrasias and advanced cancers. They do not transform into tumors of the blood-forming tissues.

LYMPHOGRANULOMATOSIS (HODGKIN'S LYMPHOMA) – 4845714 – tumors of the lymph nodes with the presence of Sternberg cells, of unknown etiology.

MYELOCYTOSIS (LEUKEMIA, CHRONIC MYELOID) – 5142357 – excessive number of myelocytes in the blood.

NEUTROPENIA, CONGENITAL – 8432145 – a group of rare hereditary diseases characterized by abnormally low neutrophils (white blood cells), occurs chronically or in oscillating cycles (cyclic neutropenia). See also: Agranulocytosis.

OVALOCYTOSIS, HEREDITARY (ELLIPTOCYTOSIS, HEREDITARY) – 51454323 – an inherited blood disorder in which there is a large amount of elliptical red blood cells in the blood, sometimes with clinically significant hemolysis.

PARAPROTEINEMIA PRODUCING TUMORS – 8432184 – a particular group of tumors of the lymph system including lymphoma of B-cell type, multiple myeloma, plasmocytoma, non-Hodgkin lymphoma producing abnormal immunoglobulins.

PAROXYSMAL NOCTURNAL HEMOGLOBINURIA (PNH) – 5481455 – a rare form of an acquired hemolytic anemia resulting in intravascular hemolysis, hemosiderinuria, and suppression of granulocytopoesis and thrombocytopoesis.

RADIATION SICKNESS, ACUTE – 481543294 – occurring after short-term exposure (up to a period of several days) to large doses of ionizing radiation of a greater portion of the body and leading to the death of primarily dividing cells.

RADIATION SICKNESS, CHRONIC – 4812453 – a disorder caused by the repeated exposure of the organism to radiation in small doses, which surpass a total of 100 rad (radiation absorbed dose).

01   **STOMATOCYTOSIS, HEREDITARY** – 4814581 – inheri-
02 ted autosomal dominant disease of the red blood cells causing
03 hemolytic anemia.
04
05   **THALASSEMIA** – 7765437 – a group of acquired hemo-
06 lytic anemias characterized by an excessive hypochromia
07 of the red blood cells concurrent with normal or raised iron
08 levels in the blood serum.
09
10   **THROMBOCYTOPATHY** – 5418541 – any disorder of
11 blood coagulation that results from congenital or acquired
12 dysfunction of the platelets.
13
14   **THROMBOPHILIA, HEMATOGENOUS** – 4814543 –
15 increased risk of developing recurring thromboses (blood
16 clots) primarily in the veins due to an abnormality in the sys-
17 tem of coagulation.
18
19
20
21
22
23
24
25
26
27
28
29
30
31
32
33
34

CHAPTER 11

ENDOCRINE AND METABOLIC DISORDERS – 1823451

ACROMEGALY – 1854321 – excess of growth hormone (somatotropin) resulting in bone overgrowth and soft tissue thickening, increased dimension of the peripheral parts and organs.

ADDISON'S DISEASE (ADRENAL INSUFFICIENCY) – 4812314 – a syndrome caused primarily by a disturbance of the adrenal cortex and secondarily through changes caused by a reduced secretion of the adrenocorticotropic hormone (ACTH).

CUSHING'S SYNDROME – 54321458 – excessive production of glucocortoid cortisol due to derangement of the body's hypothalamic-pituitary-adrenal axis.

DIABETES INSIPIDUS – 4818888 – commonly caused by a deficient amount of vasopressin (hypothalamic-pituitary axis dysfunction) resulting in extreme thirst and urination (polydipsia and polyuria).

DIABETES MELLITUS – 8819977 – a metabolic disorder, which results from failure of the pancreas to produce insulin and is characterized by deficient metabolism of carbohydrates resulting in hyperglycemia, sugar in the urine and other metabolic disturbances.

01   **DYSPITUITARISM, PUBERAL JUVENILE DYSPITUI-**
02 **TARISM SYNDROME** – 4145412 – dysfunction of the hypo-
03 thalamic-pituitary axis with increased secretion of growth
04 hormone, adrenocorticotropic hormone, thyrotropin, and
05 gonadotropin.
06
07   **GENDER DIFFERENTIATION, CONGENITAL DISOR-**
08 **DERS OF** – 5451432 – an illness arising from chromosomal
09 abnormalities.
10
11   **GOITER, ENDEMIC** – 5432178 – non-toxic swelling of
12 the thyroid gland common in areas, which have soil with an
13 iodine deficiency.
14
15   **GOITER, TOXIC DIFFUSE (GRAVES' DISEASE)** –
16 5143218 – a condition characterized by an overactive and
17 enlarged thyroid gland.
18
19   **GROWTH HORMONE DEFICIENCY (HYPOPHYSEAL**
20 **DWARFISM)** – 4141414 – a condition characterized by stun-
21 ted growth through lack of growth hormone.
22
23   **HYPERINSULINEMIA (DYSINSULINISM)** – 48454322
24 – caused by overproduction of insulin resulting in hypoglyce-
25 mia attacks. The cause could be found in hormone producing
26 tumors such as the Islet of Langerhans tumor (insulinoma) or
27 diffuse hyperplasia of pancreatic beta cells.
28
29   **HYPERPROLACTINEMIA** – 4812454 – excess secretion
30 of prolactin, a syndrome with amenorrhea and galactorrhea in
31 women and hypogonadism in men.
32
33   **HYPOGONADISM (MALE)** – 48143121 – pathologically
34 decreased production of sex hormones (androgenes).

HYPOPARATHYROIDISM (PARATHYROID TETANY) – 4514321 – a disease characterized by a reduced functionality of the parathyroid glands, increased neuro-muscular excitability and muscular spasms.

HYPOPITUITARISM (PANHYPOPITUITARISM, SIMMOND'S DISEASE) – 48143214 – chronic dysfunction of the hypothalamic-pituitary axis with secondary hypofunction of the peripheral adrenal glands.

HYPOTHYROIDISM (MYXEDEMA) – 4812415 – a condition that develops when the thyroid gland is underactive.

OBESITY – 4812412 – overweight, excessive body mass due to accumulation of fatty tissue.

OSTEITIS FIBROSA CYSTICA – 5481412 – a disease of unknown etiology marked by overactivity of the parathyroid glands.

PHEOCHROMOCYTOMA – 4818145 – neuroendocrine tumor, benign or malignant, originating in the chromaffin cells of the medulla of the adrenal glands or in the extra-adrenal tissue

SEXUAL DEVELOPMENT, PREMATURE – 4814312 – when any signs of sexual development occur under the age of eight in a girl and under the age of ten in a boy.

THYROIDITIS – 4811111 – inflammation of the thyroid gland. The inflammation of a diffuse enlarged thyroid is called strumitis.

TUMORS (SEE ALSO: ACROMEGALY, VIRILISM, HYPERINSULINEMIA, HYPERPARATHYROIDISM,

01 **PHEOCHROMOCYTOMA)** – 4541548 – endocrine disorders
02 of a tumorous nature.
03
04   **VIRILISM** – 89143212 – development of male secondary
05 characteristics in a woman caused by elevation of male hor-
06 mones in the female organism.
07
08
09
10
11
12
13
14
15
16
17
18
19
20
21
22
23
24
25
26
27
28
29
30
31
32
33
34

CHAPTER 12

OCCUPATIONAL DISEASES – 4185481

OCCUPATIONAL DISEASES, CAUSED BY CHEMICAL AGENTS – 9916515 – diseases caused by exposure to hazardous chemicals.

OCCUPATIONAL DISEASES, EXPOSURE TO PHYSICAL FACTORS (VIBRATION DISEASE) – 4514541 – a vibrational disorder caused by the long-term effect (at least 3 to 5 years) of vibrations in a production environment (machinery).

OCCUPATIONAL DISEASES, THROUGH THE INFLUENCE OF BIOLOGICAL AGENTS – 81432184 – see Chpt 14: *Infectious Diseases*.

OCCUPATIONAL DISEASES, THROUGH THE OVEREXERTION OF INDIVIDUAL ORGANS AND SYSTEMS – 4814542 – diseases caused by chronic functional overexertion, microtraumatizing, and the effect of rapid, repetitive movements (repetitive strain injury).

CHAPTER 13

ACUTE TOXICATION – 4185412

ACUTE POISONINGS – Contact poisoning – 4814823 – toxic substances absorbed by the skin.

– INGESTED POISONS – 5142154 – conditions caused by the ingestion of endogenous and exogenous substances through the mouth.

– INHALED POISONS – 4548142 – intake of toxic substances into the body through breathing.

– INJECTED POISONS – 4818142 – intoxication after injection of medications in a toxic dose or by insertion of toxic substances into a body orifice (anus, vagina, ear canal).

– POISONING CAUSED BY SNAKEBITES AND OTHER POISONOUS ARTHROPODS (INSECTS, SPIDERS, CRABS, SCORPIONS, TICKS, ETC.) – 4812521.

– SCORPION STINGS – 4188888 – acute, severe pain locally at the puncture site. The pain often radiates out over the branches of the nervous system.

– SNAKEBITES – 4114111 – acute poisoning caused by the venom of a snake.

– **TARANTULA SPIDER BITES** – 8181818 – this bite usually does not produce a serious local reaction, but it may trigger an allergic reaction with symptoms like rash, breathing difficulty and collapse and general malaise.

– **WASP AND BEE STINGS** – 9189189 – these stings are accompanied by acute, severe pain. Hyperemia and edema occur in the region of the sting.

EXOTOXIC SHOCK – 4185421 – failure of the cardiovascular system caused by the release of toxins into the bloodstream.

KIDNEY DAMAGE (TOXIC NEPHROPATHY) – 5412123 – from exposure to nephrotoxic substances (antifreeze, mercuric chloride, dichloroethane, carbon tetrachloride among others).

LIVER DAMAGE (HEPATOPATHY, TOXIC) – 48145428 – resulting from ingestion or inhalation of hepatotoxic substances (dichloroethane, carbon tetrachloride as well as some poisonous plant substances and medications such as Danabol).

PSYCHONEUROTIC DISORDER FROM TOXIC EXPOSURE – 9977881 – disorders of a psychological, neurological and physical nature caused by a combination of direct intoxication of various structures of the central and peripheral nervous systems (exogenous toxicosis) that results in a secondary intoxication of other organs and systems, particularly the liver and the kidneys (endogenous toxicosis).

CHAPTER 14

INFECTIOUS DISEASES – 5421427

ALVEOLOCOCCOSIS (ALVEOLAR ECHINOCOCCO-SIS, SMALL FOX TAPEWORM) – 5481454 – Pathogen: maggot stage of the bandworm, Echinoccus multilocularis.

AMOEBIASIS – 1289145 – a gastrointestinal infection caused by the protozoan parasite Entamoeba histolytica and marked by dysentery and ulcerative lesions of the colon. Sometimes complications occur in form of liver abscesses and damage to the lung and other organs.

ANKYLOSTOMIASIS (HOOKWORM INFESTATION) – 4815454 – caused by two parasitic nematodes, which attach themselves to the duodenum and jejunum.

ANTHRAX – 9998991 – an acute disease that affects the skin, lungs and intestines; may develop into septic shock.

ASCARIASIS (ROUNDWORM INFESTATION) – 4814812 – caused by the parasitic roundworm Ascaris lumbricoides; the larvae mature in the small intestine.

BALANTIDIASIS – 1543218 – a protozoan infection caused by Balantidium coli and marked by colon ulceration and serious complications.

BOTKIN'S DISEASE – 5412514 – see *Hepatitis, viral A and B.*

BOTULISM, FOODBORNE – 5481252 – ingestion of toxin from improperly preserved or canned food.

BRILL-ZINSSER DISEASE – 514854299 – a delayed relapse of epidemic typhus years after the first infection.

BRUCELLOSIS (BANG'S DISEASE, MALTA FEVER) – 4122222 – zoonosis caused by various species of the Brucella bacteria.

CAMPYLOBACTER JEJUNI – 4815421 – a zoonotic contagious campylobacter infection marked by diarrhea, abdominal pain and malaise.

CAT SCRATCH DISEASE (LYMPHADENITIS, SUBACUTE REGIONAL) – 48145421 – an acute disease caused by contact with infected cats (bites, scratches or saliva).

CHOLERA – 4891491 – an acute infectious disease with fecal-oral transmission by the bacterium Vibrio cholerae.

CLONORCHIASIS (CHINESE LIVER FLUKE) – 5412348 – a worm infestation by the Chinese liver fluke, Clonorchis sinensis, in the class of Trematodes (flukes).

CYSTICERCOSIS – 4512824 – infestation by the pork tapeworm Cysticercus. Humans become infected by the larval stage when eating contaminated food or from human feces. Humans are the end host of the larval stage. If the pork tapeworm larvae move out of the intestine, they cause local growths and damage in the tissues (brain, eye, heart). See also: *Taeniasis.*

DIPHTHERIA – 5556679 – an acute contagious disease transmitted mainly through respiratory droplets with toxic affliction of the heart, nervous system, local affliction of mucous membranes with thick gray covering (fibrinous pseudomembrane).

DIPHYLLOBOTHRIASIS (FISH OR BROAD TAPEWORM INFESTATION) – 4812354 – infestation by the fish or broad tapeworm.

DYSENTERY (SHIGELLOSIS) – 4812148 – infection caused by Shigella bacteria; food-borne illness, transmission via fecal-oral route.

E. COLI BACTERIOSIS (ESCHERICHIOSIS) – 1238888 – gastroenteritis, urinary tract infections, hemorrhagic syndrome, etc. caused by diverse virulent strains of enteropathogenic intestinal bacteria (e.g. E. coli).

ECHINOCOCCOSIS – 5481235 – larval stages of a tapeworm parasite of the genus Echinococcus, which settles in the liver, lung and other organs and can cause cysts to form.

ENCEPHALITIS, TICK-BORNE – 7891010 – an acute viral infection that attacks the central nervous system and is marked by inflammation and damage of the grey matter of the brain and spinal cord.

ENTEROBIASIS – 5123542 – Pathogen: the pinworm, Enterobius, which parasitizes in parts of the small intestine and colon.

ENTEROVIRUSES – 8123456 – a non-specific febrile illness with flu-like symptoms (summer cold) caused by enterovirus infection and marked by muscle ache, gastrointestinal symptoms, and symptoms of the central nervous system and the skin.

ERYSIPELAS – 4123548 – an acute bacterial (streptococcus) infection marked by recurrent, painful inflammation of sharply defined areas of the skin with fever and general malaise.

FASCIOLIOSIS (FASCIOLIASIS) – 4812542 – parasitic infestation with the liver fluke Fasciola hepatica or Fasciola gigantica.

FOOD POISONING – 5184231 – a food-borne illness caused by bacterial toxins resulting from the consumption of food or water contaminated by various microorganisms and their pathogenic toxins.

FOOT AND MOUTH DISEASE – 9912399 – an acute viral disease marked by fever, general malaise, painful sores, damage to the mucous membranes of the mouth and to the skin in the region of the hands (skin rash blisters).

GIARDIASIS (LAMBLIASIS) – 5189148 – infection with Giardia lamblia marked by disturbances of the gastrointestinal tract, diarrhea, nausea; can sometimes also be asymptomatic.

HELMINTHIASIS – 5124548 – a disease caused by parasitic infestation of the organism with worms such as hookworm, ascariasis, filariasis.

HEMORRHAGIC FEVER WITH RENAL SYNDROME – 5124567 – an acute viral disease marked by dramatic nephrotic syndrome and hemorrhagic phenomena, shock and renal failure.

01   **HEPATITIS, VIRAL, A AND B (BOTKIN'S DISEASE)** –
02 5412514 – an acute infectious disease caused by the hepati-
03 tis A/B virus; transmitted by contaminated food or water (A)
04 and infectious blood or body fluid (B); leads to liver damage,
05 jaundice, and general malaise. See also Chpt 8: Diseases of
06 the Digestive System, Hepatitis, acute – 58432141.
07
08   **HERPES SIMPLEX** – 2312489 – a viral disease caused by
09 the herpes simplex virus, affects the skin and mucosa leading
10 sometimes to keratoconjunctivitis also affecting the organs
11 and the central nervous system.
12
13   **HUMAN IMMUNODEFICIENCY VIRUS (HIV, AIDS)** –
14 5148555 – characterized by a long incubation period with
15 progressive failure of the immune system resulting in oppor-
16 tunistic infections (viral, bacterial, protozoal, fungal) and
17 malignancies that are lethal.
18
19   **HYDROPHOBIA** – 4812543 – see *Rabies*.
20
21   **HYMENOLEPIASIS (DWARF TAPEWORM INFESTA-**
22 **TION)** – 54812548 – infestation by the dwarf tapeworm.
23
24   **INFLUENZA, SEASONAL (FLU)** – 4814212 – an acute
25 viral disease spread by airborne droplets.
26
27   **LEGIONELLOSIS (LEGIONNAIRES' DISEASE)** –
28 5142122 – an acute infectious disease caused by bacteria of
29 the species Legionella and marked by fever, general malaise,
30 respiratory illness and in the severe form pneumonia, damage
31 to the gastrointestinal tract and the central nervous system.
32
33   **LEISHMANIASIS** – 5184321 – a parasitic disease caused
34 by protozoa of the genus Leishmania.

LEPROSY – 148543294 – see Chpt 21: *Skin and Venereal Diseases, Leprosy.*

LEPTOSPIROSIS (CANICOLA FEVER, WEIL'S DISEASE) – 5128432 – a bacterial zoonotic disease caused by Spirochaetes of the species Leptospira.

LISTERIOSIS – 5812438 – a zoonotic bacterial infection caused by eating food contaminated by the bacteria Disteria; multiple clinical symptoms.

LYSSA – 4812543 – see *Rabies.*

MALARIA – 5189999 – a parasitic, mosquito-borne infection with plasmodium marked by cycles of chills and fevers, anemia, enlarged liver and spleen.

MARBURG VIRUS DISEASE (MARBURG HEMORRHA-GIC FEVER, EBOLA) – 5184599 – an acute viral disease with a dramatic outbreak marked by high fatalities, hemorrhagic manifestations and damage to the liver, gastrointestinal tract and central nervous system.

MENINGOCOCCAL INFECTION – 5891423 – a bacterial infection caused by the bacterium Neisseria meningitidis leading to nasopharyngitis, meningococcal meningitis and meningococcemia (sepsis).

METAGONIMIASIS – 54812541 – an intestinal fluke caused by Trematode Metagonimus, which attaches itself to the wall of the small intestine; also a parasite of dogs, cats and pigs.

MONONUCLEOSIS, INFECTIOUS (PFEIFFER'S DISEASE, KISSING DISEASE) – 5142548 – caused by the

01 Epstein-Barr virus and marked by atypical, large lymphocy-
02 tes, an increased number of white blood cells and enlarge-
03 ment of the lymph nodes, spleen and liver.
04
05   **MYCOPLASMA INFECTION (PNEUMONIA, ATYPI-**
06 **CAL; PNEUMONIA, WALKING)** – 5481111 – an infection
07 caused by mycoplasma organisms with flu-like symptoms
08 and atypical (walking) pneumonia or infections of the genital
09 tract.
10
11   **OPISTHORCHIASIS** – 5124542 – Pathogen: the liver
12 fluke, which parasitizes the liver, the biliary passages and the
13 pancreatic duct in humans, dogs, cats and other animals.
14
15   **ORNITHOSIS (PSITTACOSIS)** – 5812435 – a disease due
16 to a Chlamydia strain contracted from birds and marked by
17 fever, cough, pneumonia, and an enlarged liver and spleen.
18
19   **PARAPERTUSSIS** – 2222221 – uncommon illness caused
20 by the Bordetella parapertussis bacterium with symptoms
21 similar to those of Pertussis but milder.
22
23   **PAROTITIS EPIDEMICA (MUMPS)** – 3218421 – a com-
24 mon acute, infectious viral childhood disease (under 15 years
25 of age) with painful swelling of the salivary glands, orchitis
26 and sometimes serous meningitis.
27
28   **PEDICULOSIS (LICE, INFESTATION OF)** – 48148121
29 – infestation of lice, blood-feeding ectoparasitic insects that
30 live on the surface of the host.
31
32   **PERTUSSIS (WHOOPING COUGH)** – 4812548 – a highly
33 contagious bacterial disease spread by droplet transmission
34 marked by coughing spells ending with a high-pitched whoop.

01   **PLAGUE** – 8998888 – an acute and highly contagious
02 disease caused by Yersinia pestis.
03
04   **Q-FEVER** – 5148542 – a zoonotic disease caused the bac-
05 teria Coxiella burnetii of the species Rickettsia and characte-
06 rized by fever, general malaise, and often damage to the lung.
07
08   **RABIES (HYDROPHOBIA, LYSSA)** – 4812543 – a viral
09 disease transmitted by the bite (saliva) of infected animals.
10
11   **ROTAVIRUS** – 5148567 – an acute viral disease mostly
12 among children; common cause of severe diarrhea.
13
14   **RUBELLA (GERMAN MEASLES)** – 4218547 – an acute
15 viral childhood disease spread by droplet transmission and
16 marked by low grade fever, swelling of the cervical and occi-
17 pital lymph nodes and pink, measles-like rash.
18
19   **RUBEOLA (MEASLES)** – 4214825 – an acute viral child-
20 hood disease spread by droplet transmission and marked by
21 fever, cough, runny nose, sore throat, maculopapular rash and
22 general malaise.
23
24   **SALMONELLOSIS** – 5142189 – an acute, infectious
25 food-borne disease caused by Salmonella bacteria.
26
27   **SCARLATINA (SCARLET FEVER)** – 5142485 – a serious
28 childhood disease (common age is 2-10) caused by Strepto-
29 coccus A and its toxin and spread through droplets and con-
30 tact transmission marked by fever, malaise, sore throat, and
31 rash.
32
33   **SCHISTOSOMIASIS (BILHARZIOSIS)** – 48125428 – a
34 helminthic disease, which affects mostly the urogenital tract,
colon, liver, spleen and sometimes the lung or nervous sys-

01 tem. Observed in countries with a tropical and subtropical
02 climate.
03
04   **STRONGYLOIDIASIS** – 54812527 – Pathogen: a round-
05 worm, which parasitizes in the small intestine (duodenum),
06 sometimes in the biliary duct or the pancreatic duct and in the
07 larval stage migrates through the lungs and bronchi.
08
09   **TAENIARHYNCHOSIS** – 4514444 – Pathogen: Taeniasis
10 saginata, the beef tapeworm.
11
12   **TAENIASIS** – 4855555 – Pathogen: Taeniasis solium, the
13 pork tapeworm. In the human intestine the young form of the
14 tapeworm develops into the adult tapeworm. A more severe
15 form of taeniasis is the cysticercosis. See also: *Cysticercosis.*
16
17   **TETANUS (LOCKJAW)** – 5671454 – a serious, life-thre-
18 atening infection caused by the toxin of the bacteria Clostri-
19 dium tetani and marked by severe damage to the nervous sys-
20 tem, tonic-clonic spasms, and failure of thermal regulation.
21
22   **TOXOPLASMOSIS** – 8914755 – a parasitic disease that
23 can become chronic with damage to the nervous system, heart
24 and eyes; lymphadenopathy and hepatosplenomegaly.
25
26   **TRICHINELLOSIS** – 7777778 – Pathogen: the round-
27 worm Trichinella.
28
29   **TRICHOCEPHALOSIS (TRICHURIASIS)** – 4125432 –
30 parasitic infestation with the whipworm Trichuris trichiuia
31 primarily in the large intestine.
32
33   **TRICHOSTRONGYLOSIS** – 9998888 – Infestation with
34 nematode worms from the Trichostrongulus family.

TULAREMIA – 4819489 – an acute infectious zoonotic disease.

TYPHOID and paratyphoid fever (Abdominal typhus) – 1411111 – a group of life-threatening diseases with high fever, malaise, diarrhea caused by Salmonella enterica and S. paratyphi A and B. The infection usually spreads by the fecal-oral route.

TYPHUS, EPIDEMIC – 1444444 – Rickettsia transmitted by the human body louse and marked by prolonged fever, headache, malaise, vascular collapse and damage to the central nervous system.

TYPHUS, QUEENSLAND TICK TYPHUS (SPOTTED FEVER) – 5189499 – a group of life-threatening diseases caused by ticks and marked by fever, general malaise and maculopapular rash.

UPPER RESPIRATORY TRACT INFECTION (COMMON COLD) – 48145488 – an infectious process of any of the components of the upper airways marked by general malaise and catarrhal symptoms.

VARICELLA (CHICKENPOX) – 48154215 – a highly contagious, usually benign childhood disease with pustular skin rash and fever; transmission through the air or skin contact.

VARIOLA (SMALLPOX) – 4848148 – a highly contagious viral disease caused by the Variola major virus characterized by a maculopapular rash, which scars, high fever and a high fatality rate.

VARIOLA MINOR – 4848148 – less virulent form of smallpox.

YERSINIA PSEUDOTUBERCULOSIS – 514854212 – an acute infectious zoonotic disease marked by fever, general malaise, and damage to the small intestine and liver; not uncommonly accompanied by a rash like in scarlet fever.

YERSINIOSIS – 5123851 – an infectious disease contracted through the consumption of undercooked meat.

CHAPTER 15

VITAMIN DEFICIENCY DISEASES – 1234895

AVITAMINOSIS – 5451234 – a group of diseases caused by chronic or long-term vitamin deficiency due to a lack in supply or a defect in metabolic assimilation. See also: *Hypovitaminosis*.

HYPOVITAMINOSIS – 5154231 – a group of diseases caused by chronic or long-term vitamin deficiency due to a lack in supply or a defect in metabolic assimilation. See also: *Avitaminosis*.

POLYAVITAMINOSIS – 4815432 – a condition caused by the deficiency of more than one vitamin.

VITAMIN A DEFICIENCY (RETINOL DEFICIENCY) – 4154812 – occurs when failing to eat sufficient amounts of Vitamin A and beta-carotene or from malabsorption in the intestines or dysfunction of synthesis from carotene.

VITAMIN B1 DEFICIENCY (THIAMINE DEFICIENCY) – 1234578 – the lack of this vitamin leads to Beriberi and to polyneuritis caused by alimentary deficiency of vitamin B1 in rice (often found in Southeast Asia where rice is the main foodstuff). A frequent cause is impaired nutrition from chronic diarrhea, persistent vomiting or malabsorption.

VITAMIN B2 DEFICIENCY (RIBOFLAVIN DEFICI-ENCY) – 1485421 – results from malnutrition or conditions of insufficient absorption from intestine or dysfunction of its phosphorylation or elevated excretion.

VITAMIN B3 DEFICIENCY (VITAMIN PP DEFICIENCY, NIACIN DEFICIENCY) – 1842157 – caused by an insufficient supply of this vitamin in the diet (particularly where maize is the main foodstuff), from poor diet or as the result of disorders that affect its absorption (diarrhea, alcoholism). Higher intake is needed during pregnancy or physical strain.

VITAMIN B6 DEFICIENCY (PYRIDOXINE DEFICI-ENCY) – 9785621 – caused in adults by the suppression of the healthy gut flora by drug interaction (pyridoxine-inactivating drugs), long-term consumption of antibiotics, tuberculostatic medication and sulfonamides, and especially in times of increased need of this vitamin (pregnancy, extreme physical strain).

VITAMIN C DEFICIENCY (ASCORBIC ACID DEFICI-ENCY) – 4141255.

VITAMIN D DEFICIENCY – 5421432 – much importance is attributed to the deficiency of ergocalciferol D2 and cholecalciferol D3.

VITAMIN K DEFICIENCY – 4845414 – seldom occurring in adults, Vitamin K deficiency is due to poor absorption because of obstruction or compression of the bile ducts that prevent the bile salts, which are needed for the intestinal absorption of phylloquinone, from going into the intestines (see Chpt 8: *Disorders of the Digestive Organs, Malabsorption*).

CHAPTER 16

DISEASES IN CHILDHOOD - 18543218

ADRENAL HYPERPLASIA, CONGENITAL – 45143213 – a congenital, autosomal recessive disease caused by a disorder of the steroid production leading to virilization.

ALLERGIC DIATHESIS (PREDISPOSITION TO ALLERGIES) – 0195451 – an inherited predisposition of the organism to allergic diseases.

ALLERGIES, RESPIRATORY – 45143212 – a group of diseases with damage to the air passages due to allergen exposure.

ALPHA 1-ANTITRYPSIN DEFICIENCY – 1454545 – leads to accumulation of abnormal protein in the liver resulting in impaired liver function and damage.

ANEMIA – 48543212 – see Chpt 10: *Blood Diseases.*

ANEMIA, IRON DEFICIENCY – 1458421 – various conditions lead to iron deficiency: prematurity (lower newborn iron stores), food related or impaired intestinal absorption of iron.

ANEMIA, TOXIC HEMOLYTIC – 45481424 – caused by accidental poisonings (nitrofurantoin, sulfonamid = sulfa drugs, anilin color, derivatives of nitrobenzol, and naphthalene.

01   **ASTHMA BRONCHIALE** – 58145428 – allergic disease
02 marked by periodic attacks with shortness of breath, whee-
03 zing caused by spasms (bronchospasm), edema of the bron-
04 chial wall and increased mucus production.
05
06   **BRONCHITIS, ACUTE** – 5482145 – inflammation of
07 varied origins of the trachea, bronchi and bronchioles.
08
09   **BRONCHITIS, ALLERGIC** – 5481432 – characterized by
10 repeated relapses with a stubborn penetrating cough coming
11 often in attacks and mainly in the night. During auscultation
12 non-resonating, wet crackles can be heard in the lungs in
13 addition to the wheezing. There is no expiratory dyspnea.
14
15   **CELIAC DISEASE** – 4154548 – atrophy of the mucosa of
16 the small intestine and malabsorption.
17
18   **CRAMPS (SPASMS)** – 51245424 – involuntary, tonic,
19 unpleasant or painful contractions of a muscle group of vary-
20 ing intensity, length and extent.
21
22   **CYSTIC FIBROSIS (MUCOVISCIDOSIS)** – 9154321 – a
23 recessive genetic disorder affecting the exocrine glands resul-
24 ting in excessively sticky mucus, which causes chronic lung
25 infections, pancreas and intestinal dysfunction and less com-
26 monly liver and kidney problems, and salty sweat.
27
28   **DE TONI–DEBRÉ–FANKONI SYNDROME** – 4514848
29 – marked by osteomalacia similar to (hypophosphatemic)
30 rickets, but in distinction to phosphate diabetes accompanied
31 by a number of severe general symptoms such as failure to
32 thrive and high susceptibility to infections.
33
34   **DIABETES INSIPIDUS** – 5121111 – a congenital disease
in which the renal tubular collecting ducts are unable to con-

01 centrate urine in response to ADH (vasopressin) or there is a
02 defect in ADH production.

04   **DIABETES MELLITUS** – 4851421 – absolute or relative
05 insulin deficiency resulting in a dysfunction of the carbohy-
06 drate metabolism with hyperglycemia and glucosuria (eleva-
07 ted sugar in the blood and urine) as well as other metabolic
08 disturbances.

10   **DIABETES, PHOSPHATE** – 5148432 – occurs when the
11 kidney fails to resorb phosphate leading to phosphaturia,
12 low phosphate in the blood and linked to Vitamin D resistant
13 rickets.

15   **DYSPEPSIA, PARENTERAL** – 8124321 – a dyspepsia
16 that occurs as a side effect and is related to infections or con-
17 ditions outside of the stomach and intestinal tract (respiratory
18 infections, otitis, urinary tract infection).

20   **DYSPEPSIA, SIMPLE** – 5142188 – an acute disorder
21 of the digestive system caused by nutritional mistakes such
22 as overfeeding, the ingestion of foodstuffs that exceed the
23 digestive capacity and functions of the system (e.g. artificial
24 feeding), ending breastfeeding in the summertime, or over-
25 heating.

27   **DYSPEPSIA, TOXIC** – 514218821 – a serious acute dis-
28 ruption of the digestion accompanied by extreme disturban-
29 ces of the metabolic processes.

31   **DYSTONIA,   VEGETATIVE-CIRCULATORY**   –
32 514218838 – often observed in preadolescence and puberty
33 and frequently with a genetic predisposition, caused by
34 chronic intoxications, over-exhaustion, long-term emotional
stress leading to lethargy and weakness.

EXUDATIVE ENTEROPATHY (ENTEROPATHY, PRO-TEIN-LOSING) – 4548123 – a group of disorders marked by excessive loss of protein (albumin) through the walls of the stomach and small intestines leading to edema, hypoproteine-mia, lowered immunity and a failure to thrive.

FETAL ALCOHOL SYNDROME – 4845421 – caused by excessive maternal consumption of alcohol before and during pregnancy resulting to various degrees in a change of the phy-sical features and developmental disabilities.

FOREIGN OBJECT ASPIRATION (CHOKING) – 4821543 – Aspiration of organic and non-organic foreign objects (Foreign object lodged in the larynx or trachea).

GALACTOSEMIA – 48125421 – a genetic disorder in which there is a defect in the metabolism of galactose (galac-tose-glucose conversion).

GLOMERULONEPHRITIS, IN CHILDREN – 5145488 – an infectious allergic disease of the kidneys.

HEART DEFECTS, CONGENITAL – 14891548 – etio-logy unknown as for the entire group of congenital defects. It is assumed that incomplete or abnormal development of the heart occurs in the third to the eighth week of pregnancy. This can be caused especially by the rubella virus (German meas-les) or parotitis virus (mumps) during pregnancy.

HEMOLYTIC DISEASE OF THE NEWBORN (RHESUS DISEASE, ERYTHROBLASTOSIS FETALIS) – 5125432 – hemolysis leads to neonatal jaundice due to antibodies made by the mother directed against the red blood cells of the fetus and to Rhesus incompatibility.

HEMOPHILIA – 548214514 – a hereditary, recessive x-linked disorder.

HEMORRHAGIC DIATHESIS – 0480421 – see also *Purpura rheumatica, Hemophilia.*

HEMORRHAGIC DISEASE OF THE NEWBORN – 5128543 – due to disturbances of the coagulation mechanism.

HEPATITIS – see Chpt 8: *Disorders of the Digestive Organs.*

HISTIOCYTOSIS, X-TYPE – 5484321 – a group of rare diseases in which excessive numbers of histiocytes form tumors and are affecting various parts of the body.

HYPERVITAMINOSIS D – 5148547 – a condition occurring after over-dosing with Vitamin D or through increased sensitivity to Vitamin D.

HYPOTHYROIDISM – 4512333 – decreased functioning of the thyroid gland.

INFANTILE TETANY (SPASMOPHILIA) – 5148999 – a disorder in infants and small children marked by the tendency to involuntary muscle contractions (tonic spasms) due to hypocalcemia (low calcium).

INTRACRANIAL BIRTH TRAUMA – 518999981 – damage to the brain of the child during birth due to intracranial hemorrhage.

JAUNDICE, NEONATAL (ICTERUS NEONATORUM) – 4815457 – see also *Hemolytic disease of the newborn.*

01   **LARYNGITIS, ALLERGIC** – 58143214 – occurs often in
02 infants. The course of the illness can often be recurrent and
03 periodically accompanied by a "barking" cough and hoarse-
04 ness.
05
06   **LEUKEMIA** – 5481347 – see Chpt 10: *Blood Diseases.*
07
08   **LYMPHATIC PREDISPOSITION** – 5148548 – a congeni-
09 tal insufficiency of the lymph system accompanied by redu-
10 ced functioning of the thymus, the main organ controlling
11 maturation of the lymphocytes.
12
13   **MALABSORPTION SYNDROME** – 4518999 – impaired
14 intestinal absorption through the mucosa of the small intes-
15 tine of one or several nutrients and particularly in conditions
16 of vitamin deficiency.
17
18   **NEPHRITIS, HEREDITARY (ALPORT SYNDROME)**
19 – 5854312 – etiology unknown but a genetic mutation is
20 suspected. Affected is the protein structure of the basement
21 membranes in the kidney and other organs.
22
23   **PHENYLKETONURIA** – 5148321 – a congenital genetic
24 disorder that damages the central nervous system and leads to
25 severe mental retardation.
26
27   **PNEUMONIA, CHRONIC** – 51421543 – a chronic infec-
28 tion that forms in infants due to a congenital abnormality of
29 the bronchopulmonary system and other inherited diseases
30 (Bronchopulmonary dysplasia).
31
32   **PNEUMONIA, INTERSTITIAL** – 4814489 – see Chpt 7:
33 *Respiratory Diseases, Pneumonia.*
34

PNEUMONIA, NEONATAL – 5151421 – infection of the lung in a newborn.

PNEUMONITIS, HYPERSENSITIVE (ALLERGIC ALVE-OLITIS) – 51843215 – inflammation of the alveoli in the lung caused by allergy inhaled organic allergens (dust, molds).

POLYARTHRITIS, CHRONIC UNSPECIFIED – 8914201 – see Chpt 6: *Rheumatic Diseases, Arthritis, rheumatoid.*

PORTAL HYPERTENSION – 45143211 – occurs with any type of chronic liver disease (cirrhosis) or with an extrahepatic cause like splenic vein thrombophlebitis. Occurs often in children who have had umbilical sepsis as newborns or have a congenital malformation of the portal vein.

PSEUDOCROUP – 5148523 – See *Laryngitis, subglottic.*

PSEUDOCROUP (LARYNGITIS, SUBGLOTTIC; LARYNGOTRACHEOBRONCHITIS) – 1489542 – an acute infection of the larynx and trachea with swelling causing obstruction of the respiratory passages.

PURPURA RHEUMATICA (HENOCH-SCHOENLEIN PURPURA, SCHOENLEIN-HENOCH PURPURA) – 5128421 – a small vessel vasculitis with small hemorrhages under the skin creating the characteristic purpura, sometimes accompanied by abdominal pain and pain and swelling of the joints.

PYLORIC STENOSIS (INFANTILE HYPERTROPHIC PYLORIC STENOSIS) – 5154321 – see *Surgeries in Childhood.*

PYLOROSPASM – 5141482 – vomiting starting early after birth, less persistent and less violent contractions than with pyloric stenosis.

RENAL DIABETES (RENAL GLUCOSURIA) – 5142585 – a congenital defect in the function of the tubules that are responsible for glucose resorption.

RENAL SALT-WASTING SYNDROME (PSEUDOHYPO-ALDOSTERONISM) – 3245678 – salt wasting syndrome of the kidney due to insensitivity of the tubular system to aldosterone, often observed after pyelonephritis (mimics hypoaldosteronism).

RESPIRATORY DISTRESS SYNDROME IN NEWBORNS – 5148284 – non-infectious, pathological process in the lungs that forms in the prenatal and early neonatal periods of the infant and appears as respiratory disturbances.

RHEUMATIC HEART DISEASE – 5481543 – See Chpt 6: *Rheumatic Diseases, Rheumatic heart disease.*

RHINITIS UND SINUSITIS, ALLERGIC – 5814325 – appears often in children from 2 to 4 years of age. The two conditions seldom occur isolated and combine with damage to the trachea and in the mouth and throat and sometimes also in the auditory canal and middle ear.

RICKETS, (VITAMIN D DEFICIENCY, RACHITIS) – 5481232 – a Vitamin D deficiency of exogenous or endogenous origin. See also Chpt 15: *Vitamin Deficiency Diseases, Vitamin D deficiency.*

SEPSIS, NEONATORUM – 4514821 – a serious (dramatic) invasive, infectious disease (often bacterial).

STAPHYLOCOCCUS INFECTION – 5189542 – a widespread acute and chronic infection caused by the Staphylococcus species.

SUBFEBRILE CONDITION IN CHILDREN – 5128514 – a condition with multiple causes such as chronic infections (tonsillitis, adenoiditis, etc.) or concomitant chronic diseases (tuberculous intoxication, lymphogranulomatosis, etc.).

SUBSEPSIS ALLERGICA (WISSLER'S SYNDROME) – 5421238 – a rheumatic disease of possibly allergic origin affecting children and adolescents.

TOXIC SYNDROME (TOXICOSIS WITH EXSICCOSIS) – 5148256 – a severe general and unspecific reaction of the organism of the young child to the invasion of microbial toxins, viruses and nutrients of poor quality.

TRACHEITIS, ALLERGIC – 514854218 – recurrent attacks of a stubborn cough coming mainly in the night disturbing the child's sleep.

TUBERCULOSIS – 5148214 – a infectious disease caused by the acid-fast Mycobacterium tuberculosis that affects mainly the lungs, intestines, bones, joints, skin and eyes.

TUBERCULOSIS, LATENT (TUBERCULOSIS, ASYMPTOMATIC; TUBERCULOSIS, SILENT) – 1284345 – an asymptomatic primary tuberculosis with TB skin reactivity in the absence of clinical or significant x-ray findings.

VOMITING – 1454215 – occurs especially often in children and more frequently the younger the child. With babies, vomiting occurs as a result of overfeeding (habitual vomiting, regurgitation). Vomiting often accompanies febrile diseases in children and

01 infants and more seldom also older children. In periods of fever
02 vomiting is not necessarily caused directly by the condition, but
03 can also be the result of an unsuitable diet or the ingestion of medi-
04 cations (especially with antipyretic medicines or sulfonamides).
05
06 ## SURGICAL CONDITIONS
07 ## IN CHILDREN – 5182314
08
09   This chapter covers the most important and serious surgi-
10 cal conditions in children.
11
12   **ANGIOMA (HEMANGIOMA)** – 4812599 – a congenital,
13 benign tumor of small blood vessels.
14
15   **APPENDICITIS, CHILDHOOD** – 9999911 – in contrast
16 to adults in children the symptoms develop more rapidly and
17 they tend to develop peritonitis.
18
19   **ATRESIA AND STENOSIS, DUODENAL** – 5557777 – a
20 partial or complete mechanical obstruction of the duodenum.
21
22   **ATRESIA, ANAL AND RECTAL** – 6555557 – an inheri-
23 ted, complete closure of the anus and rectum.
24
25   **ATRESIA, BILIARY** – 9191918 – congenital malforma-
26 tion of the bile ducts inside and/or outside of the liver.
27
28   **ATRESIA, ESOPHAGEAL** – 8194321 – congenital clo-
29 sure of the esophagus.
30
31   **ATRESIA, SMALL INTESTINE** – 9188888 – an inherited
32 complete closure of the small intestine.
33
34   **CEPHALOHEMATOMA (SUBPERIOSTAL HEMOR-
RHAGE)** – 48543214 – a soft hematoma between the peri-

osteum and the skull, most frequently located at the parietal bones, that occurs during childbirth.

ESOPHAGUS, CHEMICAL BURN OF – 5148599 – damage to the esophagus through acid or alkaline substances.

HEMORRHAGE, GASTROINTESTINAL – 5121432 – the mucous membranes (diapedesis bleeding), erosions, and ulcers among other sources can be the cause of the bleeding.

HERNIA, DIAPHRAGMATIC – 5189412 – a defect in the diaphragm that allows the abdominal organs to move up into the chest cavities. See also Chpt 16: *Surgical Diseases of the Thorax Organs: Hernia, congenital diaphragmatic* – 518543257.

INVAGINATION – 5148231 – an intestinal obstruction caused by the infolding of one part of the intestine within another and which is often the cause of ileus in children.

MECKEL'S DIVERTICULUM – 4815475 – a congenital outpouching (diverticulum) from the wall of the small intestine that forms as a remnant of the omphalomesenteric duct.

OMPHALOCELE (AMNIOCELE) – 5143248 – congenital incomplete closing of the umbilical ring after birth, abdominal contents protrude through the defect covered only by a thin membrane (amniotic sac).

OSTEOMYELITIS, EPIPHYSEAL – 12345895 – inflammation of bone tissue with abscess cavities in the epiphysis.

PALATOSCHISIS (CLEFT PALATE) – 5151515 – a congenital birth defect of the palate.

01   **PHLEGMON, NEWBORNS** – 51485433 – a spreading,
02 diffuse purulent inflammation in the soft or connective tissue
03 leading to skin necrosis.
04
05   **PYLORIC STENOSIS** – 5154321 – a form of gastric out-
06 let obstruction occurring in infants and caused by hypertro-
07 phy of the pyloric muscles resulting in forceful vomiting in
08 the first few months in infancy.
09
10   **TERATOMA,   SACROCOCCYGEAL   REGION   –
11 481543238 – a tumor composed of tissues not normally pre-
12 sent at the site.
13
14
15
16
17
18
19
20
21
22
23
24
25
26
27
28
29
30
31
32
33
34

CHAPTER 17

OBSTETRICS, GYNECOLOGICAL DISORDERS – 1489145

AMNIOTIC FLUID EMBOLISM – 5123412 – a medical emergency in which the amniotic fluid enters into the bloodstream of the mother and triggers an allergic reaction resulting in cardiogenic shock and respiratory failure.

ASPHYXIA, PERINATAL – 4812348 – caused by the decrease or lack of oxygen in the organism culminating in non-oxidized metabolic products in the blood.

HEMORRHAGE, DURING CHILDBIRTH – 4814821 –hemorrhage during labor and hemorrhage following childbirth.

LABOR, ABNORMAL PATTERNS DURING – 14891543 – poor uterine contraction strength, slow progress of labor, overly strong labor activity and abnormal labor patterns belong to the main types.

MILK GLANDS, DYSFUNCTION OF DURING LACTATION PERIOD – 48123147 – decreased secretion of milk (hypogalactia).

MOLE, HYDATIDIFORM – 4121543 – abnormal growth of chorionic tissue around an aborting embryo creating fluid-filled sacs in the uterus.

PAIN MANAGEMENT DURING CHILDBIRTH – 5421555 – physical, emotional and mental preparation for childbirth to reduce negative emotions and anxiety and to increase confidence in the ability to adapt to labor and to take an active role in the birthing process.

PELVIS, NARROW – 2148543 – differentiated into an anatomically narrow pelvis or a clinically (functionally) narrow pelvis.

PELVIS, NARROW (ANATOMICALLY) – 4812312 – when one of the dimensions of the pelvis is reduced by 1.5 to 2 cm.

PELVIS, NARROW (CLINICALLY) – 4858543 – this condition can occur with an anatomically narrow pelvis and also with a normally sized pelvis, but with a large fetus, or with an abnormal position of the fetus (asynclitic birth, face presentation, head in posterior position).

PLACENTA PRAEVIA – 1481855 – the placenta is attached to the uterine wall close to or covering the cervix opening.

PLACENTAL ABRUPTION – 1111155 – caused by disorder vascular diseases in the mother (severe toxemia of pregnancy, hypertension, nephritis, etc.), inflammatory and dystrophic changes of the uterus, degenerative changes to the placenta (prolonged pregnancy, hypovitaminosis), or increased uterine distension (excess of amniotic fluid, multiple pregnancy, large fetus).

POLYHYDRAMNIOS (HYDRAMNIOS) – 5123481 – an excess of fluid in the amniotic sac (more than 2 liters).

POSTNATAL/POSTPARTUM PERIOD, NORMAL – 12891451 – normally lasts 6 to 8 weeks.

POSTPARTUM COMPLICATIONS – 41854218 – distention of the uterus with retained lochia (lochiometra) caused by retroversion (tilting) of the uterus due to a lengthy bed period or the uterus not returning to its normal size.

PREGNANCY, BIRTH AND DUE DATE (FOR A NORMAL PREGNANCY WITH A NORMAL DUE DATE) – 1888711 – the date of the last menstruation as well as the date of the first movements of the fetus and the results of external examination of the pregnant woman are used to determine the due date.

PREGNANCY, ECTOPIC (FOR THE RESTORATION OF HEALTH AND RETENTION OF THE FETUS) – 4812311 – positioning and development of the fertilized egg outside of the womb (in 99% of the cases in the fallopian tubes).

PREGNANCY, MULTIPLE (PREGNANCY WITH TWO OR MORE FETUSES) – 123457854.

PREGNANCY, POST-TERM (PROLONGED) – 5142148 – an extended pregnancy (beyond 42 weeks).

PREGNANCY, UTERINE – 1899911 – a normal pregnancy lasting 280 days or 40 weeks dated from the last menstrual period.

PRETERM BIRTH – 1284321 – birth between the 28th to the 39th week of pregnancy.

TEARS IN EXTERNAL GENITALS DURING CHILDBIRTH – 148543291 – tears in the area of the vulva and in the

mucous membranes of the urethra opening (urethral rupture)
and the clitoris, often accompanied by severe bleeding.

TOXEMIA, IN PREGNANCY (PRE-ECLAMPSIA) –
1848542 – abnormal conditions in pregnancy: toxicity, gestosis (vomiting that arises in pregnancy and generally disappears after delivery), salivation, edema, jaundice, asthma bronchiale. See also Chpt 9: Diseases of the Kidneys and Urinary Tract, Renal eclampsia.

UMBILICAL CORD WOUND CARE FOR NEWBORNS –
0123455 –the umbilical wound is often the entry point for infections. An infection can lead to a sepsis. Special care is important in the treatment of the umbilical cord (aseptic and antiseptic treatment).

UMBILICAL CORD, PROLAPSE – 1485432 – protrusion of the umbilical cord occurring in breech delivery, transverse position or with a narrow pelvis.

GYNECOLOGICAL DISORDERS – 1854312

ADNEXITIS – see *Oophoritis, Salpingitis.*

ADRENOGENITAL SYNDROME – 148542121 – marked by excessive production of adrenocortical hormones (androgens) leading to virilization.

AMENORRHEA – 514354832 – absence of menstrual period for 6 months or more.

ANOVULATORY CYCLE – 4813542 – menstrual cycle with absence of ovulation and luteal phase.

BARTHOLINITIS – 58143215 – inflammation of the Bartholin's gland at the entry of the vagina.

CANCER, VULVA – 5148945 – a malignant epithelial tumor, and rarely as cylindrical cell cancer.

CERVICAL EROSION (ECTROPION, CERVICAL) – 54321459 – a change of the squamous cells into columnar cells caused by tear, injury during childbirth or abortion.

CHORIONEPITHELIOMA (CHORIOCARCINOMA) – 4854123 – a rare malignant tumor that develops in the tissues of the reproductive system.

COLPITIS – 5148533 – see *Vaginitis*.

CYST, OVARIAN – 5148538 – fluid-filled sacs within an ovary.

CYSTADENOMA, OVARIAN – 58432143 – a benign cystic tumor of the ovary.

DYSMENORRHEA – 4815812 – pain during menstruation.

ENDOCERVICITIS – 4857148 – an inflammation affecting both the endometrium (inner lining of the uterus) and the uterine cervical canal.

ENDOMETRIOSIS – 5481489 – heterotopia of the endometrium (inner lining of the uterus).

ENDOMETRITIS – 8142522 – inflammation of the inner lining of the uterus.

GONORRHEA – 5148314 – a sexually transmitted disease caused by Neissenia gonorrhoeae.

HEMORRHAGE, DYSFUNCTIONAL BLEEDING OF THE UTERUS – 4853541 – a dysfunctional condition of the uterus caused by an imbalance in the production of the sex hormones of the ovary.

INFERTILITY (STERILITY) – 9918755 – inability to conceive (after two years or longer) in women who lead a normal sex life without contraception.

KRAUROSIS VULVAE – 58143218 – a precancerous condition of the vulva marked by dystrophic, atrophic and sclerotic changes of the skin.

LEUKOPLAKIA, VULVA OR CERVIX – 5185321 – a precancerous condition of the vulva or cervix marked by hyperkeratosis and parakeratosis with further sclerotic development and marked by the appearance of white blotches that cannot be dabbed off.

LEUKORRHEA (VAGINAL DISCHARGE) – 5128999 – a common condition marked by a quantitative or qualitative alteration of the vaginal secretion.

MENOPAUSE (CLIMACTERIC) – 4851548 – physical, emotional and mental changes accompanying the end of the fertile phase of a woman's life.

MYOMA, UTERINE – 51843216 – a benign tumor of the uterus originating in the smooth muscle tissue.

OOPHORITIS (ADNEXITIS) – 5143548 – inflammation of an ovary, often combined with inflammation of the fallopian tubes (see Salpingitis).

OVARIAN APOPLEXY (CORPUS LUTEUM RUPTURE) – 1238543 – hemorrhage into the ovary with bleeding into the abdomen caused in most cases by a rupture of the corpus luteum.

PARAMETRITIS – 5143215 – inflammation of the connective tissue around the uterus.

POLYCYSTIC OVARIAN DISEASE (STEIN-LEVENTHAL SYNDROME) – 518543248 – a disturbance of the hypothalamic-pituitary axis caused by dysfunction of the adrenal glands or primary impairment of the ovaries.

POLYP, CERVICAL OR UTERINE – 518999973 – benign overgrowth of the endometrium near the cervical opening, possibly caused by chronic inflammation and vice versa.

PREMENSTRUAL SYNDROME (PMS) – 9917891 – a functional disruption of the nervous system, the circulatory system and the endocrine system in the second half of the menstrual cycle.

PROLAPSE, UTERUS AND VAGINA – 514832183 – occurs mostly in advanced years due to trauma during labor, heavy work shortly after delivery or with involution processes of the genitals; typical in older women.

PRURITUS VULVAE (VULVA, ITCHY) – 5414845 – itchy vulva, could be precancerous (Paget's disease).

SALPINGITIS – 5148914 – inflammation of a fallopian tube.

01   **TUBERCULOSIS, GENITAL** – 8431485 – a secondary
02 disease caused by spreading infection from the primary loca-
03 tion (lungs) through a hematogenous route or via the lympha-
04 tic system from mesenteric lymph nodes and the peritoneum.
05
06   **VAGINITIS (COLPITIS)** – 5148533 – inflammation of the
07 mucous membrane of the vagina.
08
09   **VULVITIS** – 5185432 – inflammation of the external
10 genitals, often combined with vaginitis.
11
12   **VULVOVAGINITIS** – 5814513 – inflammation of the
13 vagina and the external genitals.
14
15
16
17
18
19
20
21
22
23
24
25
26
27
28
29
30
31
32
33
34

CHAPTER 18

NEUROLOGICAL DISEASES – 148543293

ABSCESS, CEREBRAL – 1894811 – the collection of pus within the brain tissue.

ADIE SYNDROME (MYDRIASIS, PUPILLOTONIA) – 18543211 – damage to the innervation of the pupil of the eye with one-sided dilated pupil (mydriasis) and pupillotonia.

AMYOTROPHIC LATERAL SCLEROSIS (MOTOR NEURON DISEASE, LOU GEHRIG'S DISEASE) – 5148910 – progressive neurodegenerative disease caused by degeneration of the upper and lower motor neurons resulting in muscle atrophy, spasm and bulbar symptoms.

ANEURYSM, CEREBRAL – 1485999 – a localized dilation of a cerebral artery or vein. The most common location is in the network of blood vessels at the base of the brain called the Circle of Willis.

ARACHNOIDITIS – 4567549 – a serous inflammation of the arachnoid membrane that encloses the brain and spinal cord.

ASTHENIA (CHRONIC FATIGUE SYNDROME) – 1891013 – marked by listlessness, a tendency to fatigue and loss of strength to face physical or emotional challenges.

ATHETOSIS – 1454891 – constant slow, involuntary, repetitive writhing movements.

BRAIN INJURY, TRAUMATIC – 51843213 – mechanical trauma to the head with temporary or permanent damage to the brain.

CEREBRAL PALSY – 4818521 – a group of motor disorders (non-progressive impairment of the motor development) related to brain injury that occurred during fetal development or birth.

CHARCOT-MARIE-TOOTH DISEASE – 4814512 – an inherited neurological disorder that is characterized by slowly progressive atrophy of the feet and legs with loss of touch sensation.

CHOREA – 4831485 – hyperkinetic, involuntary movements, especially of the upper extremities, the body and the face.

COMA – 1111012 – a state of unconsciousness resulting from a dysfunction of the brain stem.

DIENCEPHALIC SYNDROME (HYPOTHALAMIC SYNDROME) – 514854215 – a complex of symptoms related to lesions of the hypothalamic area in the diencephalon.

ENCEPHALITIS, VIRAL – 48188884 – an acute inflammation of the brain caused by a neurotropic virus.

EPIDURITIS – 888888149 – a collection of pus that forms on the dura mater of the brain or spinal cord.

EPILEPSY – 1484855 – a chronic neurological disorder marked by episodes of recurrent seizures accompanied by complex clinical and paraclinical symptoms.

FUNICULAR MYELITIS (PUTNAM-DANA SYN-DROME) – 518543251 – a subacute combined degeneration of the posterior and lateral columns of the spinal cord often due to a B12 deficiency.

HEADACHE (CEPHALGIA) – 4818543 – often a symptom of an underlying medical condition.

HEADACHE, CLUSTER – 4851485 – a paroxysmal attack (several bouts a day) of excruciating unilateral pain, orbital, supraorbital or temporal.

HEPATOCEREBRAL DYSTROPHY (WILSON'S DISEASE, HEPATOLENTICULAR DEGENERATION) – 48143212 – an autosomal recessive, genetic disorder of the copper metabolism occurring usually between the ages of 10 to 35 and marked by progressive impairment of the liver and the subcortical ganglia.

HERPES ZOSTER (SHINGLES) – 51454322 – a varicella-zoster virus infection of a spinal root ganglion with dermatomal distribution of severe pain and a vesicular rash.

HYDROCEPHALUS – 81432143 – an abnormal accumulation of cerebrospinal fluid in the ventricles of the brain leading to dilation of the ventricles and compression of the brain.

MENINGITIS – 51485431 – inflammation of the membranes of the spinal cord or brain.

MIGRAINE – 4831421 – a paroxysmal one-sided headache accompanied by nausea and vomiting.

MONONEUROPATHY – 4541421 – damage of a single nerve or nerve group.

MULTIPLE SCLEROSIS – 51843218 – a relapsing, debilitating neurological disorder that damages the myelin sheath (demyelination) in the white matter areas of the brain and spinal cord leading possibly to glial scarring.

MUSCULAR DYSTROPHY, PROGRESSIVE – 85432183 – an inherited, progressive muscular disorder leading to weakness, degeneration and dystrophy of the skeletal muscles.

MYASTHENIA GRAVIS – 9987542 – a chronic neuromuscular disease marked by varying degrees of weakness of the skeletal muscles of the body.

MYELITIS – 4891543 – inflammation of the gray and white matter of the spinal cord. With transverse myelitis the inflammation is restricted to the segments involved.

MYELOPATHIA – 51843219 – pathology of the spinal cord due to chronic processes such as tumors or vascular or degenerative disease.

MYOTONIA CONGENITA (THOMSEN'S DISEASE) – 4848514 – an inherited, autosomal dominant disease with severe myotonia, cramps with muscle stiffness and pain that affects the voluntary muscles.

MYOTONIC DYSTROPHY (CURSCHMANN-BATTEN-STEINER SYNDROME) – 481543244 – marked by myotonia, muscular atrophy and endocrine dysfunction. The muscular atrophy attacks mainly the face and neck. Other developments include cataracts, alopecia, testicular atrophy, and decreased IgG levels.

NARCOLEPSY – 48543216 – attacks of excessive daytime sleepiness and falling asleep at inappropriate times. Cataplexy and sudden muscular weakness may be experienced.

NEUROPATHY, FACIAL NERVES – 518999955 – caused by otitis, fractures of the temporal bone or tumors in the region of the cerebellopontine angle (acoustic neuroma).

NEURORHEUMATISM – 8185432 – rheumatic lesions of the nervous system.

NEUROSYPHILIS – 5482148 – an infection of the central nervous system coming often many years after the initial infection with syphilis.

OPHTHALMOPLEGIA – 4848532 – paralysis of one or more extraocular muscles, sometimes in combination with iris sphincter palsy.

PARALYSIS, FAMILIAL PERIODIC – 5123488 – an inherited, rare disorder marked by episodes of flaccid paralysis of the extremities.

PARKINSON'S DISEASE (PARKINSONISM) – 54811421 – chronic degenerative disorder of the nervous system caused by a defect of the dopamine metabolism in the subcortical ganglia showing symptoms such as tremor, rigidity and loss of motion.

01   **PHAKOMATOSES** – 5142314 – a group of disorders of
02 the central nervous system combined with skin and/or eye
03 lesions (retinal angiomatosis).
04
05   **POLIOMYELITIS (PARALYSIS, INFANTILE)** – 2223214
06 – an acute viral, infectious disease most commonly with viral
07 invasion of the motor neurons of the anterior horn cells in the
08 spinal column and the lower motor neurons and marked by
09 the development of flaccid paralysis, areflexia and atrophy.
10
11   **POLYNEUROPATHY** – 4838514 – damage to diverse
12 peripheral nerves with symmetrical motor and sensory
13 involvement, flaccid paralysis distally in the legs and occasi-
14 onal damage to the cranial nerves.
15
16   **POLYNEUROPATHY, ACUTE INFLAMMATORY**
17 **DEMYELINATING (GUILLAIN-BARRÉ SYNDROME)** –
18 4548128 – a peripheral nerve disorder and autoimmune
19 disease leading to demyelinisation of the nerve roots.
20
21   **POST-LUMBAR PUNCTURE SYNDROME** – 818543231
22 – development of headaches and symptoms like meningism
23 after a lumbar puncture.
24
25   **RADICULOPATHY (RADICULITIS, SCIATICA)** –
26 5481321 – a painful condition with motoric or autonomic
27 dysfunction caused by compression of the nerve roots through
28 spinal disc herniation or osteochondrosis.
29
30   **SLEEP DISORDER** – 514248538 – sleeping disorders
31 accompanied by hypersomnia (excessive sleepiness). See
32 also *Narcolepsy.*
33
34   **SPINAL AMYOTROPHY** – 5483312 – a group of hereditary chronic diseases marked by progressive muscle atrophy

and paralysis caused by degradation of the anterior horn cells of the spinal cord.

SPINAL APOPLEXY (SPINAL INSULT) – 8888881 – acute disruption of the blood supply in the spinal cord.

STROKE (APOPLEXY, CEREBROVASCULAR INSULT, SPINAL STROKE SYNDROME) – 4818542 – a cerebralvascular accident due to ischemia or hemorrhage.

SYNCOPE (FAINTING SPELLS) – 4854548 – sudden loss of consciousness most commonly due to a sudden lack of oxygen to the brain often vasovagal (orthostatic hypotension) or because of cardiac dysfunction.

SYRINGOMYELIA – 1777771 – a chronic disease marked by the development of cavities within the spinal cord and medulla oblongata causing pain and weakness but also leads to a loss of pain and temperature sensation.

TREMOR – **3148567** – involuntary, rhythmic muscle movements resulting from either alternating or synchronous contractions of reciprocally innervated antagonist muscles.

TRIGEMINAL NEURALGIA – 5148485 – brief and intense pain attacks along the distribution of the branches of the trigeminal nerve.

TUMOR, BRAIN – 5451214 – neoplasm of the brain, destroys brain cells and increases the pressure within the skull.

TUMOR, BRAIN AND SPINAL CORD – 5431547 – See Chpt 2: *Tumors, Tumor, brain and spinal cord.*

01   **TUMOR, PERIPHERAL NERVOUS SYSTEM** –
02 514832182 – mostly neurinomas, often present in neurofib-
03 romatosis type 1.
04
05   **TUMOR, SPINAL CORD** – 51843210 – neoplasms loca-
06 ted in the spinal cord that are mostly metastases from primary
07 cancers elsewhere.
08
09   **VERTIGO, CEREBRAL (DIZZINESS)** – 514854217 –
10 sensation of a patient of turning within himself or of the sur-
11 rounding objects and the feeling of falling or of the ground
12 being instable and pulling out from under one's feet (sinking
13 through the floor).
14
15
16
17
18
19
20
21
22
23
24
25
26
27
28
29
30
31
32
33
34

CHAPTER 19

PSYCHIATRIC DISORDERS – 8345444

AFFECTIVE DISORDER – 548142182 – includes the bipolar disorder of depression and mania. The depressive syndrome is marked by bad moods and longings, sometimes with the feeling of physical pressure in the thorax and intellectual and motor inhibitions; the manic syndrome by a pathological euphoria combined with extreme optimism.

ALCOHOLISM – 148543292 – the disease develops with chronic ethanol intoxication leading to a pathological, uncontrollable addiction to alcoholic drinks accompanied by alcohol withdrawal syndrome, disruption of mental abilities, somatic and neurological disorders and lowering of the ability to work and of social standards.

BIPOLAR DISORDER (MANIC-DEPRESSIVE DISORDER) – 514218857 – a condition marked by episodes of mania and depression usually separated by times of a normal state of mind.

CATATONIA – 51843214 – a disorder marked by changes in muscle tone, a deficit of motor activity (movement) and stupor and excitement, often alternating.

DELUSIONAL DISORDER – 8142351 – a delusion is an absolute, uncorrected opinion created through pathological causes and lacking any adequate external foundation.

ENCEPHALOPATHY, POST-TRAUMATIC – 18543217 – includes a complex of neurological, physiological and mental-emotional dysfunction arising after repeated head injury in the past.

GRANDIOSITY – 148454283 – pathological condition in which a person exaggerates their talents, capacity and achievements in an unrealistic way.

HALLUCINOSIS – 4815428 – a condition caused by a profusion of hallucinations that arises over a longer period of time and is present even without a disturbance of consciousness.

HYPOCHONDRIA – 1488588 – preoccupation with one's health and concern at even the smallest discomfort; convinced he has a serious illness.

HYSTERICAL SYNDROME – 5154891 – unmanageable emotional excess arising mostly in extreme stress or conflict situations.

KORSAKOFF'S SYNDROME – 4185432 – a symptom complex of anterograde and retrograde amnesia marked by memory deficit for actual events.

MENTAL CONFUSION – 4518533 – pathological confusion usually refers to a loss of orientation sometimes accompanied by disordered consciousness and memory along with a loss of self-confidence.

NARCOMANIA (ADDICTION TO NARCOTICS) – 5333353 – a state of periodic or chronic intoxication produced by the repeated consumption of a drug (natural or synthetic) and marked by a "need (compulsion) to continue taking the drug and to obtain it by any means; a tendency to increase the dose; a psychic (psychological) and generally a physical dependence on the effects of the drug; and detrimental effects on the individual and on society" (WHO).

NARCOMANIA AND TOXICOMANIA – 1414551 – diseases caused by the addiction to (narcotic) substances, which produce intoxication.

NEGATIVE (DEFICIT) SYMPTOMS – 5418538 – a mental state characterized by a lack of emotions, interest and responsiveness, often associated with schizophrenia leading to an inability to carry out daily routines.

NEUROTIC DISORDER – 48154211 – one of the most common psychogenic reactions marked by distress whereby behavior is not outside socially acceptable norms.

OBSESSIVE COMPULSIVE DISORDER (FIXED IDEAS) – 8142543 – marked by uncontrollable obsessive thoughts, ideas and compulsive behaviors.

OLIGOPHRENIA (MENTAL RETARDATION) – 1857422 – congenital or early acquired feeblemindedness marked by an underdevelopment of intelligence.

PARALYSIS, PROGRESSIVE – 512143223 – a late latent, diffuse syphilitic, psychopathological and mental and neurological disturbance ending in progressive dementia.

PSYCHIC DEFECT – 8885512 – a defective, negative condition marked by the pathological absence of certain mental processes and leading to dissociation (breakdown of integrating activity).

PSYCHOORGANIC SYNDROME – 51843212 – a condition of mental debility caused by organic brain disorders.

PSYCHOPATHIC DISORDER (ANTISOCIAL PERSONA- LITY DISORDER) – 4182546 – a stabile, congenital mental state of the personality that prevents complete adaptation to social standards.

PSYCHOSES, SYMPTOMATIC – 8148581 – includes mental disturbances arising from pathological conditions, diseases of the inner organs, infectious diseases and endocrine disorders.

PSYCHOSIS, PRESENILE (PSYCHOSIS, INVOLUTIO- NAL) – 18543219 – a group of psychic disorders that manifest at a time of regression (54 to 60 years old) and take either the form of depression or that of delusion of a paranoid or paraphrenic nature.

PSYCHOSIS, REACTIVE – 0101255 – marked by the connection of the disease with some psychological trauma and its disappearance after the removal of the cause.

PSYCHOSIS, SENILE – 481854383 – occurs in old age and includes senile dementia and other forms of senile psychosis.

PSYCHOTIC DISORDER, SUBSTANCE-INDUCED – 1142351 – caused by acute or chronic exposure to toxins through industrial, nutritional or chemical substances kept in the house or through drugs or medications.

SCHIZOPHRENIA – 1858541 – a chronic progressive, pathological and disabling mental illness that gradually changes the personality.

CHAPTER 20

SEXUAL DISORDERS – 1456891

EJACULATION DISORDERS – 1482541 – possibly caused by prostatic congestion near the urethra or the para-central lobules syndrome.

ERECTILE DYSFUNCTION – 184854281 – appears during disorders of the spinal cord, cauda equina syndrome, penile nerve disorders (induratio penis plastica), injury, tumors or toxicity.

FRIGIDITY, FEMALE – 5148222 – loss or total lack of sexual desire, lack of sexual arousal and orgasm.

HYPERSEXUALITY – 5414855 – excessive sexual drive, normal for certain age periods.

IMPOTENCE – 8851464 – inability to achieve or sustain an erection and thus disrupting normal sexual intercourse.

ONANISM (MASTURBATION) – 0021421 – self-stimulation of the erogenous zones to achieve orgasm.

PSYCHOSEXUAL DISORDER (SEXUAL PERVERSION) – 0001112 – pathological disorders in the attainment of sexual arousal or the conditions of satisfaction.

01 **SEXUAL DYSFUNCTION** – 1818191 – difficulty in expe-
02 riencing sexual excitement (from lack of desire to problema-
03 tic erection, ejaculation and orgasm) and relating to adapta-
04 tion in intimacy.
05
06 **SEXUAL DYSFUNCTION, FROM NEUROENDOCRINE**
07 **DISORDERS** – 1888991 – due to damage in the diencephalon
08 (area of the hypothalamus and pituitary gland) or in specific
09 sex hormone producing glands (adrenals, gonads).
10
11 **SEXUAL DYSFUNCTION, IMAGINARY** – 1484811 –
12 marked by difficulties in sexual performance that are not phy-
13 siological and not based in age or the constitutional norm or
14 abnormalities of sexual identity.
15
16 **SEXUAL DYSFUNCTION, PSYCHIC** – 2148222 – often
17 occurring as multiple disorders caused by psychogenic fac-
18 tors.
19
20 **VAGINISMUS** – 5142388 – involuntary spasms of the
21 muscles surrounding the vagina and pelvic floor during inter-
22 course or gynecological exam.
23
24
25
26
27
28
29
30
31
32
33
34

CHAPTER 21

DERMATOLOGICAL AND VENEREAL DISEASES – 18584321

ACNE VULGARIS – 514832185 – occurs most commonly during puberty and is characterized by inflammatory, purulent damage to the sebaceous glands during seborrhea.

ACTINOMYCOSIS OF THE SKIN – 148542156 – most common form of the bacterial pseudomycosis.

ALOPECIA (BALDNESS, HAIR LOSS) – 5484121 – loss of hair, usually from the scalp and less frequently from other hairy parts of the body.

BALANOPOSTHITIS – 5814231 – inflammation of the foreskin (prepuce) and the head of the penis (glans).

CANDIDIASIS (THRUSH, YEAST INFECTION) – 9876591 – a fungal infection of the skin and mucous membranes with a variety of clinical forms, caused by yeast (Candida species).

CONDYLOMA ACUMINATUM (FIG WARTS, GENITAL WARTS) – 1489543 – marked by genital warts, figwarts, wart-like papillomas and sometimes the development of a fleshy growth.

01   **DERMATITIS** – 1853121 – an inflammatory disorder of
02 the surface of the skin caused by a reaction to external sub-
03 stances.

05   **DERMATITIS, ATOPIC (NEURODERMITIS, DIFFUSE)**
06 – 5484215 – a chronic, recurrent skin disease marked by
07 itching, red to brownish gray patches, thickening of the skin
08 (lichenification).

10   **ECZEMA** – 548132151 – a disease marked by inflamma-
11 tion of the superficial layer of the skin (dermatitis), neuro-all-
12 ergic hypersensitivity to internal or external irritants, itching
13 and a chronic-recurrent progression.

15   **ERYTHEMA MULTIFORME** – 548142137 – exhibits a
16 cyclical pattern marked by eruptions of papules, vesicles and
17 blisters on the skin and mucous membranes.

19   **ERYTHEMA NODOSUM** – 15184321 – a form of allergic
20 vasculitis with red bumps under the skin on the lower extre-
21 mities.

23   **ERYTHRASMA** – 4821521 – a widespread skin disease
24 caused by the Corynebacterium minutissimum.

26   **FAVUS** – 4851481 – dermatomycosis, a fungal disease of
27 the skin, hair and nails marked by a chronic, long-lasting pro-
28 gression.

30   **GONORRHEA, IN MEN** – 2225488 – the most common
31 sexually transmitted disease characterized by purulent ureth-
32 ritis.

34   **GONORRHEA, IN WOMEN – GONORRHEA** – see Chpt
    17: *Obstetrics, Gynecological Disorders, Gonorrhea.*

ICHTHYOSIS – 9996789 – a disorder of the skin marked by dry, thickened, scaly or flaky skin.

LEPROSY – 148543294 – chronic infectious disease.

LEUKODERMA (VITILIGO) – 4812588 – a rare skin condition of unknown etiology marked by acquired depigmentation of patches of skin and which presents cosmetic problems for the patient.

LICHEN RUBER PLANUS – 4858415 – widespread disorder of unknown etiology with damage to the skin, the mucous membranes and less frequently to the nails.

LYELL'S SYNDROME (EPIDERMAL NECROLYSES, TOXIC) – 4891521 – toxic-allergic damage to the skin and mucosa accompanied by damage to the internal organs and nervous system.

LYMPHOGRANULOMATOSIS INGUINALIS – 1482348 – a sexually transmitted bacterial disease.

MASTOCYTOSIS – 148542171 – a chronic disease affecting the skin and also the inner organs and bones.

MOLLUSCUM CONTAGIOSUM – 514321532 – a viral skin infection mostly occurring in children.

MYCOSIS FUNGOIDES – 4814588 – the most common form of cutaneous T-cell lymphoma.

NEURODERMATITIS – 1484857 – a group of very itchy skin diseases leading to scratch marks and lichenification (leathery skin patches).

PEMPHIGUS (BLISTERING DISEASE) – 8145321 – a condition of unknown etiology marked by blistering and sores (erosions) on the skin and mucous membranes with loss of cohesion between the epidermal cells (acantholysis).

PITYRIASIS ROSEA – 5148315 – a non-fungal, perhaps viral skin disorder with a characteristic rash.

PITYRIASIS VERSICOLOR – 18543214 – a slightly infectious yeast type skin fungus.

PRURIGO NODULARIS – 5189123 – a disease from the group of itchy dermatoses marked by the appearance of swollen nodules with extreme itchiness.

PRURITUS (ITCHING) – 1249812 – a condition mostly of a neuroallergic nature. Itching is differentiated as a subjective symptom (eczema, hives, scabies) and as an independent skin disease (idiopathic itching of the skin).

PSORIASIS – 999899181 – a widespread chronic, non-infectious disease with damage to the skin, the nails and the joints.

PYODERMA – 51432149 – any skin disease that is purulent.

RINGWORM (EPIDERMOPHYTON) – 5148532 – a fungal skin infection causing superficial and cutaneous mycosis.

RINGWORM (MICROSPORUM) – 1858321 – a genus of fungus that causes tinea diseases of the skin and hair (ringworm in dogs and cats).

RINGWORM (TRICHOPHYTOSIS) – 4851482 – a fungal infection of the skin, hair or nails.

ROSACEA – 518914891 – a frequent complication of seborrhea in middle-aged and older people marked by small red bumps or pustules on the face and teleangiectasia of the small blood vessels in the background.

SCABIES – 8132548 – a parasitic contagious skin infection marked by itching (pruritus) mostly at night, scabies mite trails and scratch marks.

SEBORRHEA – 1234512 – a disorder of unknown etiology that affects the sebaceous glands causing them to overproduce sebum (skin oil).

SKIN TOXICOSIS – 514832184 – toxic, adverse reactions of the skin to contact with or ingestion, inhalation or intravenous supply of toxic-allergic substances (foodstuffs, medicines, chemical agents).

STEVEN-JOHNSON SYNDROME – 9814753 – a serious, acute toxic, allergic condition with a generalized rash on the skin and mucous membranes; a severe, malignant type of erythema multiforme.

SYPHILIS (LUES) – 1484999 – primarily a sexually transmitted, infectious disease marked by a chronic-recurrent progression with damage to all organs and systems.

TRICHOPHYTON RUBRUM – 4518481 – the frequent pathogen for hand and foot mycoses, especially onychomycoses, athlete's foot and jock itch.

01   **TUBERCULOSIS, CUTANEOUS** – 148543296 – various
02 skin lesions and conditions caused by infection of the skin
03 and tissues with the Mycobacterium tuberculosis.
04
05   **TUMOR, SKIN** – 1458914 – a generic term for a group of
06 tumors originating from different parts of the epidermis.
07
08   **ULCUS MOLLE (CHANCROID, SOFT CHANCRE)** –
09 4815451 – a sexually transmitted disease marked by painful,
10 small ulcers on the genitals.
11
12   **URTICARIA (HIVES)** – 1858432 – an allergic disorder
13 marked by the formation of water blisters on the skin and
14 mucous membranes.
15
16   **VASCULITIDES, CUTANEOUS** – 5142544 – a group of
17 inflammatory, allergic dermatoses marked by damage of the
18 hypodermal blood vessels of various sites.
19
20   **VASCULITIS (ANGIITIS, CUTANEOUS)** – 1454231
21 – a group of inflammatory-allergic dermatoses marked by
22 destruction of the blood vessels.
23
24   **VERRUCAE (WARTS)** – 5148521 – a viral skin disorder
25 marked by small, hard, benign tumor-like growths of a non-
26 inflammatory nature.
27
28
29
30
31
32
33
34

CHAPTER 22

SURGICAL DISEASES – 18574321

SURGICAL DISEASES IN ADULTS – 5843215

ABDOMEN, ACUTE – 5484543 – conditions requiring urgent medical care, hospitalization and diagnosis.

ABSCESS – 8148321 – a collection of pus and dead tissue in a capsule of granulation tissue.

ACTINOMYCOSIS – 4832514 – an infectious bacterial disease caused by the Actinomyces species (common saprophyte of the oral cavity).

ANAL FISSURE – 81454321 – a longitudinal, crack-like ulcer in the mucous membrane of the anal canal most often occurring on the posterior midline.

ANEURYSM – 48543218 – bulging of the wall of a blood vessel with destruction of the wall by the inner layers (true aneurysm) or without protrusion of the inner layers but with an encapsulating covering (false aneurysm); can be positioned in the surrounding tissue or between the vessel coverings.

APPENDICITIS, ACUTE – 54321484 – a non-specific inflammation of the vermiform appendix of the cecum.

BRONCHIECTASIS – 4812578 – dilation of portions of the large bronchi or bronchioli commonly occurring in the lower left lobe.

BURNS, THERMAL – 8191111 – thermal damage caused by the effect of local high temperature (heat or fire) on the tissue.

CARBUNCLE – 483854381 – purulent inflammation of the hair follicles and the subcutaneous fat in its surroundings.

CARDIAC ANEURYSM – 9187549 – develops as a complication in myocardial infarction in 10% to 15% of the cases.

CHOLANGITIS – 8431548 – a non-specific inflammation of the bile ducts.

CHOLECYSTITIS, ACUTE – 4154382 – an acute non-specific inflammation of the gall bladder.

CHOLECYSTOLITHIASIS – 0148012 – formation of bile stones in the gall bladder, less often in the biliary or hepatic ducts.

COLITIS, ULCERATIVE – 48143211 – ulcerative lesions in the lining of the colon often occurring first in the rectum and marked by a lengthy course of the disease and severe local and systemic complications.

CONTUSION (BRUISE) – 0156912 – blunt trauma to the tissue without laceration or breaking of the skin.

CROHN'S DISEASE – 94854321 – a non-specific inflammation of the gastrointestinal tract (more often involving the terminal ileum or the proximal large intestine) and leading to the formation of inflammatory infiltrations or serpiginous linear ulcers that develop due to perforations, internal or external fistula formation or other severe complications.

CRYPTORCHIDISM – 485143287 – undescended or incomplete descension of the testicles or their malposition.

CYST, BRANCHIAL CLEFT (CYST, LATERAL NECK, PHARYNGEAL FISTULA) – 514854214 – originates from a remainder of the embryonic development of the 2nd or 3rd bronchial cleft.

CYST, BREAST (FIBROCYSTIC BREASTS) – 4851432 – most cysts are relegated to hormonal dysfunction or less frequently to retention.

CYST, THYROGLOSSAL (CYST, MEDIAN NECK) – 4548541 – median cysts and fistulas develop from embryonic remnants of the thyroglossal duct.

DECUBITUS (BED SORES) – 6743514 – a skin necrosis caused by many factors such as: unrelieved pressure, friction or shearing forces. In younger people it can be caused by spinal cord injuries, in older people often by being bedridden for lengthy periods of time.

DIVERTICULOSIS, COLON – 4851614 – these diverticles are the result of increased or abnormal pressure in the colon causing pouches in the intestinal lining and are generally caused by a weakening of the connective tissue in older age.

DIVERTICULUM – 48543217 – outpouching of the mucous membrane through a defect in the muscular tissue of a digestive tube.

01   **DUMPING SYNDROME (GASTRIC)** – 4184214 – often
02 associated with patients who have had a gastrectomy (par-
03 tial or full removal of the stomach) and often after Billroth
04 II surgery.
05
06   **ELECTRIC SHOCK INJURIES** – 5185431 – tissue
07 damage caused by electric current passing through the body
08 due to accidents at work or at home and with children.
09
10   **EMPYEMA, PLEURAL (PLEURITIS, PURULENT)** –
11 514854223 – accumulation of pus in the pleural cavity with
12 secondary compression of lung tissue.
13
14   **ENDANGIITIS OBLITERANS** – 4518521 – a widespread
15 peripheral vascular disorder of the arteries of the lower ext-
16 remities usually combined with arteriosclerosis obliterans or
17 thrombangiitis.
18
19   **FIBROADENOMA, BREAST** – 4854312 – a breast tumor
20 that appears to be hormone related (hyperestrogenic).
21
22   **FISTULA, EPITHELIAL COCCYGEAL, (CYST, PILONI-**
23 **DAL)** – 9018532 – a congenital anomaly, a remnant of faulty
24 coalescence of the cutaneous covering of the back during
25 embryonic life in the shape of tube-like indentation in the
26 perineum, which usually contains hair and skin debris.
27
28   **FISTULA, RECTAL** – 5189421 – the pathological forma-
29 tion of a pathway in the wall of the rectum (usually in the
30 area of the Crypts of Margagni) leading into a blind opening
31 (incomplete) or with both an internal and external opening
32 (complete).
33
34   **FLAT FEET (PES PLANUS, PLATYPODIA)** – 1891432 –
    partial or complete collapse of the longitudinal arch of the

foot and less frequently of the transverse arch.

FOREIGN OBJECTS, BRONCHI – 5485432 – various objects aspirated into the lower airways (sometimes also of plant or animal origin).

FOREIGN OBJECTS, ESOPHAGUS – 14854321 – accidental swallowing of objects such as coins, dentures, fishbones, chunks of meat, etc. that lodge in the esophagus.

FOREIGN OBJECTS, SOFT TISSUE – 148543297 – various objects often found on the arms or legs such as slivers of metal, glass, or wood splinters.

FOREIGN OBJECTS, STOMACH – 8184321 – Infants and people with mental illnesses can swallow knives, forks, spoons, needles, buttons, coins and other objects.

FRACTURE – 7776551 – a break in or rupture of bone tissue usually caused by trauma.

FROSTBITE – 4858514 – localized damage to skin and other tissues due to extreme cold.

FURUNCLE (BOIL) – 5148385 – a purulent inflammation of the hair follicle caused mainly by Staphylococcus.

GAS GANGRENE – 41543218 – a gas-forming, anaerobic infection causing tissue to necrotize.

GYNECOMASTIA – 4831514 – enlarged breasts in men.

HEMARTHROSIS – 4857543 – bleeding in the cavity of a joint.

HEMORRHAGE, EXTERNAL (BLEEDING, EXTERNAL) – 4321511 – bleeding through a break in the skin due to traumatic mechanical injury resulting in damaged blood vessels.

HEMORRHAGE, INTERNAL (BLEEDING, INTERNAL) – 5142543 – bleeding into an anatomical cavity or hollow organ due to damage to the blood vessels through trauma, aneurysm rupture or vessel erosion.

HEMORRHOIDS – 58143219 – varicose dilations of the venous plexus around the anus and rectum.

HERNIA – 95184321 – protrusion of intestines through a weakened spot in the abdominal wall.

HIDRADENITIS – 4851348 – a purulent inflammation of the apocrine sweat glands.

HYDROCELE, TESTIS OR SPERMATIC CORD – 481543255 – the accumulation of fluid in the scrotum around a testicle or around the spermatic cord.

ILEUS, PARALYTIC (INTESTINAL STASIS) – 4548148 – loss of bowel mobility resulting in partial or complete blockage of the small or large intestine.

INGROWN NAIL (ONYCHOCRYPTOSIS) – 4548547 – a condition where the nail grows laterally into the nail fold (the soft tissue surrounding the border of the nail).

JAUNDICE, OBSTRUCTIVE – 8012001 – cause by extrahepatic or intrahepatic obstruction of the biliary tract.

LEIOMYOMA – 55114214 – a benign tumor of a smooth muscle.

LIPOMA – 4814842 – a benign tumor composed of fatty tissue, the most common form of soft tissue tumors.

LUXATION – 5123145 – complete dislocation of a joint.

LYMPHADENITIS – 4542143 – an infection of the lymph nodes (often purulent).

LYMPHANGITIS – 484851482 – a suppurative inflammation of the lymph vessels.

MASTITIS – 8152142 – inflammation of the mammary gland.

MASTOPATHY – 84854321 – pain in the breast caused by hormonal imbalance.

MEDIASTINITIS – 4985432 – serous or purulent inflammation of the soft tissues of the mediastinum (middle part of the chest cavity between the lungs).

MEGACOLON – 4851543 – an abnormal dilation of the colon with various causes (Hirschsprung's disease, Chilaiditi syndrome, idiopathic megacolon, etc.).

MENISCUS TEAR – 8435482 – a ruptured meniscus or lesions or damage in the knee joint.

OCCLUSION OF MAJOR ARTERIES – 81543213 – acute or chronic impaired circulation in an organ caused by embolism or blood clots of a vessel (thrombosis).

ORCHIEPIDIDYMITIS – 818432151 – the non-specific inflammation of a testicle and epididymis.

OSTEOMYELITIS, TRAUMATIC – 514854221 – inflammation of bone tissue resulting from an open fracture, gunshot wounds or nearby infections.

PANCREATITIS, ACUTE – 4881431 – a disease marked by autodigestion of the pancreas and caused by activation of the pancreatic enzymes.

PARONYCHIA (PANARITIUM) – 8999999 – a non-specific inflammation of the base or side of a fingernail or a toenail.

PERITONITIS – 1428543 – an inflammation of the peritoneum often caused by a bacterial infection and more seldom through chemical inflammation due to leakage of body fluid (urine, gastric juice, bile).

PHIMOSIS, PARAPHIMOSIS – 0180010 – a condition where the prepuce (foreskin) is too tight and cannot be retracted. Paraphimosis: when the retracted foreskin cannot return to its original position.

PHLEBOTHROMBOSIS – 1454580 – the formation of a blood clot that is adherent in a vein causing partial or complete occlusion of the vessel (floating thrombus).

PHLEGMON – 48143128 – suppurative inflammation of the subcutaneous tissue with the tendency to progression.

PNEUMOTHORAX, SPONTANEOUS – 481854221 – loss of negative pressure in the pleural cavity causing partial or complete collapse of the lung.

POLYP – 4819491 – a benign tumor extending from a mucous membrane. It is either attached to the membrane by an elongated stalk or has a flat base.

POSTCHOLECYSTECTOMY SYNDROME – 4518421 – a condition after gall bladder surgery which may be described as a continuation of the symptoms which led to the surgery.

PROSTATITIS – 9718961 – inflammation of the prostate gland.

PROSTRATE ADENOMA – 51432144 – an adenomatous growth that develops from the periurethral glands of the prostrate.

PSEUDARTHROSIS – 4814214 – abnormal movement in the structural integrity of a bone resulting from inadequate healing of a fracture. See also *Traumas and Orthopedic Diseases, Pseudarthrosis* – 8214231.

PULMONARY GANGRENE – 4838543 – severe progressive putrid destruction of lung tissue because of an anaerobic infection.

PYLORIC STENOSIS – 81543211 –a disorder in the evacuation of nutriments from the stomach into the duodenum due to scarring from chronic peptic ulceration, cancer in the antrum area and less frequently to hypertrophy.

PYOPNEUMOTHORAX – 148543299 – pus, air or gas in the pleural cavity leading eventually to a collapse of the lung.

RECTAL PROLAPSE – 514832187 – a condition where the rectum wall falls out of place and protrudes through the anus.

SEBACEOUS CYST (STEATOMA) – 888888179 – a retention cyst originating from the obstruction of a sebaceous gland.

TALIPES EQUINOVARUS (CLUBFOOT) – 485143241 – a congenital foot deformity with inner rotation. The toes and bottom of the foot point inwards.

THROMBANGIITIS OBLITERANS (BUERGER'S DISEASE) – 5432142 – a systemic inflammation and clotting (thrombosis) of the arteries and veins with segmental involvement of small and medium-sized vessels and later progressing to larger vessels.

THROMBOPHLEBITIS – 1454580 – see *Phlebothrombosis.*

TORTICOLLIS (WRYNECK) – 4548512 – a stiff neck with the head tipped to the side of the affected muscle (sternocleido mastoideus) and turned facing the opposite side.

TRAUMA, INTERNAL ORGANS – 8914319 – blunt injury to the internal organs of the body.

TUBERCULOSIS, BONE – 148543281 – tuberculosis of the bones rather than of the lungs is observed in 10% of TB patients.

ULCER (STOMACH OR DUODENUM), PENETRATING – 9148532 – the penetration of an ulcer in the stomach or duodenum into adjacent organs or tissue.

ULCER, PENETRATING – 8143291 – penetration through the organ wall (stomach or duodenum) without free perforation or leakage of luminal contents into the peritoneal cavity.

ULCER, TROPHIC – 514852154 – a prolonged, non-healing tissue defect with the tendency to relapse and take a serious course.

URINARY RETENTION, ACUTE (ISCHURIA, ACUTE) – 0144444 – acute retention of urine due to enlarged prostate (adenoma), prostrate cancer, urethral stricture, bladder stones, etc.

VARICOCELE – 81432151 – a disorder of the veins around the spermatic cord marked by irregular enlargement, knotted twisting, and thinning of the walls of the veins.

VARICOSIS – 4831388 – enlarged, swollen veins in the lower extremities due to weak valves (between the deep and superficial veins) that usually prevent backflow.

WOUNDS – 5148912 – damage to the skin, usually through mechanical trauma.

ZOLLINGER-ELLISON SYNDROME – 148543295 – stomach ulceration caused by pancreatic tumors.

Surgical Diseases of the Newborn – 514218871

CHOLANGIOPATHY OF THE NEWBORN, CONGENITAL – 948514211 – an absent or blocked bile duct (biliary atresia) resulting in malfunction and liver failure.

SURGICAL DISEASES OF THE ORGANS OF THE ABDOMINAL CAVITY – 5184311 – congenital ileus (bowel obstruction); anal atresia (imperforate anus).

Surgical Diseases of the Thorax Organs – 5184312

ATRESIA, ESOPHAGUS – 518543157 – a serious birth defect formed during the embryonic period at the time the esophagus is forming and separating from the pulmonary system.

CYSTIC LUNG DISEASE, CONGENITAL – 4851484 – a malformation developing during the embryonic period in which bronchi and alveoli are created.

FISTULA, TRACHEOESOPHAGEAL – 514854714 – incomplete fusion of the tracheoesophageal folds of the primitive foregut during the embryonic period leading to a defective tracheoesophageal septum.

HERNIA, CONGENITAL DIAPHRAGMATIC – 518543257 – an intrauterine developmental defect in which abdominal organs are displaced into the chest cavity due to a defect in the diaphragm. See also Chpt 16: *Hernia, diaphragmatic* – 5189412.

PNEUMOTHORAX – 5142147 – a tear in the tissue of the lung occurring during artificial respiration.

Purulent Inflammatory Diseases – 514852171

MASTITIS, NEWBORNS – 514854238 – inflammation of the mammary glands in the newborn.

MUSCULOSKELETAL SYSTEM, DISEASES IN NEWBORNS – 514218873 – birth trauma resulting from mechanical injury, a c-section or a forceps/vacuum delivery.

OSTEOMYELITIS, ACUTE HEMATOGENOUS IN NEW-BORNS – 5141542 – a purulent septic disease in newborns.

PARAPROCTITIS, ACUTE – 4842118 – inflammation of the fatty tissue surrounding the rectum and close to the anal opening.

PERITONITIS, NEWBORNS – 4184321 – an inflammation of the peritoneum caused in newborns by a perforation of an organ wall in the digestive tract due to congenital defects in the same, by necrotizing enterocolitis and by inflammatory conditions of the organs of the abdominal cavity.

PHLEGMON, NECROTIC CUTANEOUS, IN NEW-BORNS – 514852173 – peculiar diffuse and purulent inflammation of the skin and the soft tissue that becomes necrotic in neonates (babies less than 4 weeks old).

Traumas and Orthopedic Diseases – 1418518

AMPUTATION, TRAUMATIC – 5451891 – loss of a body part, partial or whole limb, or other body parts due to mechanical force (accident).

ANKYLOSIS – 1848522 – the loss of movement or immobility of a joint due to degeneration or fusion.

BURSITIS – 75184321 – inflammation of the fluid-filled sac close to a joint.

CONTRACTURE, DUPUYTREN'S – 5185421 – a thickening of the tissue of the palm that inhibits the straightening of the fingers.

CONTRACTURE, JOINT – 8144855 – limited motion of a joint.

HALLUX VALGUS (BUNION) – 5418521 – deviation of the big toe towards the other toes, often accompanied by transverse flat feet and often occurring on both sides.

HEMARTHROSIS – 7184321 – bleeding into a joint.

PSEUDARTHROSIS – 8214231 – non-union of a fractured bone due to failure of healing and resulting in motion like a joint. See also *Surgical Diseases, Pseudarthrosis* – 8214231

SHOCK, TRAUMATIC – 1454814 – the severe general reaction of the organism to massive trauma of tissues or extreme blood loss.

SPRAINS (DISTORTION) – 5148517 – damage to muscles, tendons, and other tissues without disruption of their anatomical integrity.

TRAUMA, INNER ORGANS – 5432188 – traumatic damage to the organs of the thorax area, the abdominal cavity or the brain.

CHAPTER 23

EAR, NOSE AND THROAT DISEASES – 1851432

ABSCESS, RETROPHARYNGEAL – 1454321 – pus in the tissues and lymph nodes in the back of the throat.

ADENOIDS (TONSIL, PHARYNGEAL) – 5189514 – swelling of the lymphatic tissue in the roof of the nasopharynx.

AEROSINUSITIS (SINUS BAROTRAUMA) – 514854237 – inflammation of the sinus due to decreased barometric pressure.

ANGINA TONSILLARIS (TONSILLITIS, ACUTE) – 1999999 – an acute infectious disease with inflammation of the palatine tonsils.

ANGIOFIBROMA, NASOPHARYNGEAL JUVENILE – 1111122 – most common tumor of the nasopharynx.

ATRESIA, CHOANAL (SYNECHIA, NASAL) – 1989142 – full or partial obstruction of the nasal passage caused by (congenital) bony or soft tissue malformation.

CORYZA (RHINITIS, COMMON COLD) – 5189912 – inflammation of the mucous membranes of the nose.

DEFORMATIONS, NASAL SEPTAL – 148543285 – deformation of the nasal septum as developmental anomaly or resulting from a trauma.

EAR WAX (CERUMEN) – 48145814 – a naturally occurring substance in the ear canal.

EPISTAXIS (NOSE BLEEDS) – 65184321 – bleeding in the nose due to trauma, surgery, intranasal tumors, acute infectious diseases, hypertension, or a bleeding disorder.

EUSTACHITIS – 18554321 – inflammation of the Eustachian (auditory) tube.

FOREIGN OBJECTS, EAR – 54321545 – object in the ear. Children often place various things into the ear canal where they become lodged (paper, seed, peas, sunflower seeds, beads).

FURUNCLE, NASAL VESTIBULE – 1389145 – a result of trauma or scratching with transmission of a Staphylococcus infection by the finger of the patient.

GLOTTIS, EDEMA OF – 2314514 – the accumulation of fluid and swelling of the soft tissues, commonly in the region of the vestibular folds, subglottis or epiglottic folds.

HEMATOMA, NASAL SEPTUM – 5431482 – bleeding within the nasal septum due to trauma.

LABYRINTHITIS – 48154219 – inflammation of the inner ear that affects the vestibular and auditory system resulting in hearing problems.

LARYNGEAL WEB – 148543283 – congenital or acquired elastic membranes forming in the larynx, for example, as a reaction to chronic intubation.

LARYNGITIS – 4548511 – inflammation of the larynx.

LARYNGOSPASM – 485148248 – appears in early childhood caused by rickets, tetany, hydrocephalus or artificial feeding.

MASTOIDITIS, ACUTE – 514832186 – an acute inflammation within the mastoid, occurs often as a serious complication of purulent otitis media.

MENIERE'S DISEASE – 514854233 – a disorder of unknown etiology marked by an endolymph build-up and elevated pressure in the labyrinth.

MUCOCELE, FRONTAL SINUS (CYST, MUCOUS) – 5148322 – a cyst-like swelling or suppuration in the paranasal sinuses.

OTHEMATOMA (AURICULAR HEMATOMA, CAULIFLOWER EAR, WRESTLER'S EAR) – 4853121 – bleeding between cartilage and skin or between cartilage and the perichondrium, affecting the external ear.

OTITIS (EXTERNA, MEDIA, INTERNA) – 55184321 – inflammation in the external, middle or inner ear (see also *Labyrinthitis*).

OTOANTRITIS (MASTOIDITIS, CHRONIC) – 1844578 – inflammation of the mastoid cavity and the surrounding tissues.

OTOMYCOSIS – 514832188 – fungal ear infection of the external ear canal sometimes also affecting the eardrum.

OTOSCLEROSIS (OTOSPONGIOSIS) – 4814851 – abnormal growth of bone in the middle ear causing hearing loss, etiology unknown.

OZAENA (RHINITIS, ATROPHIC) – 514854241 – a chronic disease of the nasal cavity marked by atrophy of the mucosa and turbinate bones, crust formation and by an offensive, fetid odor.

PARALYSIS, LARYNGEAL – 1854555 – a result of inflammatory and degenerative processes in the laryngeal muscles or damage to the innervations of the laryngeal nerve.

PHARYNGITIS – 1858561 – acute or chronic inflammation of the pharynx.

PHARYNGOMYCOSIS – 1454511 – a fungal infection of the pharynx caused by Leptothrix buccalis.

POLYP, NASAL – 5519740 – a result of chronic mucosal irritation.

RHINITIS, VASOMOTOR OR ALLERGIC (POLLINOSIS, HAY FEVER) – 514852351 – sudden attacks of nasal congestion with a watery, mucus discharge and sneezing, comes as a neural response to the environment.

SCLEROMA (RHINOSCLEROMA) – 0198514 – chronic inflammation affecting the tissues of the upper respiratory tract

SEPSIS, OTOGENIC – 5900001 – the spreading of a purulent infection of the middle ear beyond the middle ear through the veins of the temporal bone or due to direct contact of the pus with the walls of the sinus sigmoideus.

SINUSITIS – 1800124 – acute or chronic inflammation of the paranasal sinuses.

STENOSIS, LARYNGEAL – 7654321 – partial or complete obstruction of the larynx, acute: croup, pseudocroup, Foreign object obstruction; chronic: inflammation, tumor, scleroma, syphilis, tumor.

STRIDOR, CONGENITAL (LARYNGOMALACIA) – 4185444 – a developmental defect of the larynx.

TINNITUS – 1488513 – inflammation of the auditory system of the inner ear.

TONSILLAR HYPERTROPHY – 4514548 – swollen tonsils, usually accompanied by hypertrophic adenoids, in childhood with enlarged lymphadenoid tissue in the pharynx.

TONSILLITIS, ACUTE – 1999999 – see *Angina tonsillaris*.

TONSILLITIS, CHRONIC – 35184321 – chronic inflammation of the palatine tonsils in adults and children.

TRAUMA, EAR – 4548515 – mechanical trauma to the ear (the most frequent form of ear damage).

TUBERCULOSIS, LARYNGEAL – 5148541 – a complication of lung tuberculosis appearing primarily in men of an age between 20 and 40 years.

01   **TUMOR, LARYNX** – 5148742 – benign lesions of the
02 larynx; common forms are polyps and papilloma.
03
04
05
06
07
08
09
10
11
12
13
14
15
16
17
18
19
20
21
22
23
24
25
26
27
28
29
30
31
32
33
34

CHAPTER 24

EYE DISEASES – 1891014

AMBLYOPIA (LAZY EYE) – 1899999 – decrease of vision in the eye without an apparent anatomical, organic problem or refractive cause.

ASTHENOPIA (EYE STRAIN) – 9814214 – eye fatigue or tiredness caused by strain.

ASTIGMATISM – 1421543 – a refraction error due to an irregular shape of the cornea or lens.

BLEPHARITIS – 5142589 – inflammation of the lid margin of the eyelids.

CATARACT – 5189142 – opacity (clouding) of the lens of the eye.

CHALAZION (EYELID CYST) – 5148582 – an eyelid cyst.

CHORIOIDITIS – 5182584 – inflammation of the vascular layer in the back of the eye (a type of uveitis), usually in combination with inflammation of the retina (chorioretinitis).

CONJUNCTIVITIS – 5184314 – inflammation of the conjunctiva (the membrane that covers the white part and the inner surface of the eye).

DACRYOCYSTITIS – 45184321 – inflammation of the lachrymal sac, often chronic.

ECTOPIA LENTIS (LENS DISPLACEMENT) – 25184321 – partial dislocation (subluxation) or complete malposition of the lens (luxation).

ECTROPION (LOWER EYELID, DROOPING) – 5142321 – an outward turning of the eyelid due to scarring occurring often after injuries, facial burns, systemic lupus erythematosus, etc., and also with age-related weakness or facial nerve palsy.

ENDOPHTHALMITIS – 514254842 – a purulent inflammation of the inner layers of the eye with formation of an abscess of the vitreous body.

EXOPHTHALMOS (PROPTOSIS, BULGING EYE) – 5454311 – the forward displacement of the eye in the orbit, protruding eyeball.

EYEBALL INJURIES – 518432118 – damage caused by blunt impact and penetrating injury from sharp objects.

GLAUCOMA (OCULAR HYPERTENSION) – 5131482 – a chronic disease of the eye with permanent or periodically increase ocular pressure, a special type of atrophy of the optic nerve, restricted visual field; differentiated into congenital, primary and secondary glaucoma.

HORDEOLUM (STYE) – 514854249 – an acute focal, purulent inflammation of the eyelid margin.

HYPEROPIA (FARSIGHTEDNESS) – 5189988 – difficulty in seeing near objects clearly while seeing distant objects clearly. The images entering the eye are focused incorrectly behind the retina.

IRITIS – 5891231 – inflammation of the iris also affecting the ciliary body (iridocyclitis).

KERATITIS – 518432114 – inflammation of the cornea.

MYOPIA (NEARSIGHTEDNESS) – 548132198 – clear vision of near objects but distant objects are blurry because the image is focused in front of the retina.

NEURITIS, OPTIC – 5451589 – caused by the spreading of an inflammation of the nasal cavities or the meninges, or an autoimmune disorder that may be triggered by infection or due to toxicity.

NYCTALOPIA (NIGHT BLINDNESS) – 5142842 – impaired vision in dim twilight or at night.

OCCLUSION, CENTRAL RETINAL ARTERY – 514852178 – obstruction of the central artery of the retina due to spasm, embolism or thrombosis.

OCCLUSION, CENTRAL RETINAL VEIN – 7777788 – obstruction of the central vein of the retina or its branches due to thrombosis or compression of a vein by thickening of the intima media.

OCULAR BURN (EYE BURN) – 8881112 – burns to the eye that are either thermal or chemical (acid, alkali, etc) in origin.

OPHTHALMIA, SYMPATHETIC – 8185321 – an injury to one eye with a resulting iridocyclitis that produces an

01 inflammation to the uninjured eye.
02
03   **OPTIC NERVE, ATROPHY** – 5182432 – degeneration of
04 the optic disk due to diseases of the optic nerve, retina, brain,
05 neurologic diseases, vascular diseases, toxicity or congenital
06 causes.
07
08   **PANOPHTHALMIA** – 5141588 – an acute, purulent
09 inflammation of the entire eye.
10
11   **PAPILLEDEMA (OPTIC DISC EDEMA)** – 145432152 – a
12 non-inflammatory swelling of the optic disc.
13
14   **PHOTO OPHTHALMIA (PHOTOKERATITIS, SNOW**
15 **BLINDNESS)** – 5841321 – burns to the conjunctiva, cornea
16 or retina due to exposure to ultraviolet light.
17
18   **PRESBYOPIA (FARSIGHTEDNESS OF THE AGING)** –
19 1481854 – an age-related process in which the eye lens loses
20 its flexibility resulting in a decrease in the ability to see near
21 objects.
22
23   **PTERYGIUM (SURFER'S EYE)** – 18543212 – a benign
24 growth of the conjunctiva extending onto the cornea.
25
26   **PTOSIS (UPPER EYELID, DROOPING)** – 18543121 –
27 can be very mild or complete with a decreased visual field.
28
29   **RETINAL DETACHMENT** – 1851760 – with no external
30 cause (primary) or due to trauma, inflammation or eye tumors
31 (secondary).
32
33   **RETINITIS** – 5484512 – inflammation of the retina.
34

01   **SCLERITIS, EPISCLERITIS** – 514854248 – inflamma-
02 tion of the sclera (the white outer coat of the eyeball) and/
03 or episclera occurring in rheumatoid arthritis, tuberculosis,
04 syphilis and less often in acute infectious diseases.
05
06   **STRABISMUS (TROPIA, CROSS-EYED SQUINT)** –
07 518543254 – an eye condition in which the optic axes diverge
08 from parallel.
09
10   **TRACHOMA** – 5189523 – a chronic, contagious infection
11 of the conjunctiva by Chlamydia trachomatis.
12
13   **ULCER, CORNEAL** – 548432194 – an open sore on the
14 cornea; infection of the erosive cornea after a traumatic break
15 through the invasion of microbes via the conjunctival sac or
16 the lachrymal duct or by microbes from the damaging object.
17
18   **UVEITIS** – 548432198 – inflammation of the uveal tract
19 structures of the eye (iris, ciliary body, choroid).
20
21   **VERNAL KERATOCONJUNCTIVITIS (CATARRH,
22 SPRING)** – 514258951 – an allergic eye condition with peri-
23 odic, seasonal (springtime) inflammation of the conjunctiva
24 or cornea with bumpy elevations under the eyelids (papillary
25 hypertrophy).
26
27
28
29
30
31
32
33
34

CHAPTER 25

DISEASES OF THE TEETH AND ORAL CAVITY – 1488514

ABSCESS, PREMAXILLARY – 518231415 – a purulent encapsulated inflammation (abscess) in the upper jaw region of the incisors.

ALVEOLITIS, DENTAL (DRY SOCKET) – 5848188 – inflammation in the socket of a tooth often occurring after the tooth has been pulled.

BLEEDING, TOOTH EXTRACTION, AFTER – 8144542 – profuse bleeding from a tooth extraction wound.

CHEILITIS (CHAPPED LIPS) – 518431482 – inflammation and cracking of the lips.

CYST, JAW – 514218877 – the pathological formation of a cavity containing fluid in a jaw.

DENTAL CALCULUS (DENTAL TARTAR) – 514852182 – hardened dental plaque composed of calcium salts.

DENTAL CARIES (TOOTH DECAY) – 5148584 – marked by progressively destructive damage to the hard tissues of the tooth.

DENTAL FOCAL INFECTION – 514854814 – a primary focus of infection, which occurs in or around a tooth (periodontal tissues) from which secondary or systemic infections can spread throughout the body.

GINGIVITIS – 548432123 – inflammation of the gum tissue.

GLOSSALGIA (TONGUE PAIN) – 514852181 – abnormal, painful sensations in the tongue (numbness, tingling, etc.).

GLOSSITIS (TONGUE INFLAMMATION) – 1484542 – a catarrhal or purulent infection of the tongue.

HYPERESTHESIA, TEETH – 1484312 – increased sensitivity to pain or touch.

HYPOPLASIA, TOOTH ENAMEL – 74854321 – the tooth enamel is deficient or defective.

JAW, FRACTURED – 5182148 – damage to the structure of the jawbone.

LEUKOPLAKIA – 485148151 – white lesions (keratosis) on the mucous membrane of the mouth caused by chronic irritation.

OSTEOMYELITIS, JAWBONE – 5414214 – a jawbone infection caused by trauma or an acute toothache involving all structures of the bone.

PAPILLITIS, INTERDENTAL – 5844522 – inflammation of the gingival papilla.

PERICORONITIS – 5188888 – inflamed or swollen gum or flap of gum tissue in the area around a partly erupted wisdom tooth.

PERIODONTAL DISEASE (PARADONTOSIS) – 58145421 – a degenerative systemic inflammation of the gum and all the deeper structures including the bone with receding gums and regression of the tooth-supporting osseous part of the bone.

PERIODONTITIS – 5182821 – inflammation of the soft tissues around the teeth leading to progressive loss of the alveolar bone around the teeth, and if left untreated, can lead to the loosening and subsequent loss of teeth.

PERIODONTITIS, APICAL – 3124601 – inflammation of the tissue around the tip of a root of a tooth. Initially caused by infection of the inner tooth pulp (from a root canal infection or a dead tooth).

PHLEGMON, MAXILLOFACIAL REGION – 5148312 – a diffuse purulent inflammation of the subcutaneous tissues in the jaw region.

PULPITIS – 1468550 – inflammation of the soft tissue (dental pulp) in the center of the tooth leading to acute attacks of pain.

STOMATITIS – 4814854 – inflammation of the mucous membrane of the mouth.

TMJ (TEMPOROMANDIBULAR JOINT), ANKYLOSIS – 514852179 – restricted motion of the TMJ resulting in difficulty in opening the mouth and impaired chewing and speech.

TMJ (TEMPOROMANDIBULAR JOINT), ARTHRITIS – 548432174 – infection and degenerative process of the TMJ.

TMJ (TEMPOROMANDIBULAR JOINT), DISLOCATION (LOCKED JAW) – 5484311 – displacement of the mandibular condyle of the TMJ.

TOOTH LUXATION – 485143277 – displacement of a tooth caused by trauma with injury to the peridontium (bone and gums that surround the tooth).

TOOTH, FRACTURED (BROKEN) – 814454251 – traumatic damage to the crown and root of a tooth.

TOOTHACHE, ACUTE – 5182544 – acute attacks of tooth pain in or around a tooth; can be mistaken as an earache or temporal pain and occurring together with inflammation of the pulp and irritated nerve roots.

XEROSTOMIA (DRY MOUTH) – 5814514 – abnormal dryness of the mouth due to lack of saliva.

01
02
03
04
05   **CHAPTER 26**
06
07   **UNKNOWN DISEASES AND CONDITIONS – 1884321**
08
09
10   In cases of unknown diseases and conditions, you should
11   base your considerations upon a division of the body into
12   seven regions: first the head, second the neck, third the right
13   hand, fourth the left hand, fifth the torso, sixth the right leg
14   and seventh the left leg.
15   Work with one or more of these regions according to need.
16
17
18
19
20   **RESTORATIVE NUMBER SEQUENCES FOR**
21   **UNKNOWN DIAGNOSES, DISEASES AND CONDITIONS**
22
23
24
25
26
27

Region	Restorative Number Sequence
Head	1819999
Neck	18548321
Right Hand	1854322
Left Hand	4851384
Torso	5185213
Right Bein	4812531
Left Bein	485148291

01
02
03
04
05
06

CHAPTER 27

ACHIEVING NORMAL
LABORATORY TEST VALUES – 1489991

07   For the restoration of deviant laboratory test values to
08 normal values, it is necessary to concentrate on the numbers,
09 which have as their goal a return to normal health within all
10 parameters. Use the same number sequences for children as
11 for adults.

12   During the concentration on the numbers of the restorative
13 number sequences in the following tables, you should take
14 into consideration that each table represents a specific per-
15 spective. This can express itself in various number sequences
16 that correlate to particular normal values.

17   The table forms what could be considered a unit or discrete
18 level of consciousness. On this level the restorative number
19 sequences, which form the table, are interconnected in their
20 contribution to building the normal values. For this reason an
21 optimal effect is achieved when, in addition to the restorative
22 number sequences you have chosen, you also concentrate on
23 all of the restorative number sequences in the table.

24   In this chapter the laboratory test values listed are those
25 normal for adults.

26

27   A number of normal laboratory test values (particularly
28 for test values used in parts of the European portion of Eura-
29 sia) have been replaced by values from unified methods. For
30 regions with extreme climatic conditions (extreme North,
31 Northeast, South) and also for the reason of genetic adap-
32
33
34

01 tation of the people of these regions to these conditions, the
02 values listed must be adjusted accordingly. All laboratory
03 values for blood tests are based upon samples taken between
04 7 and 8 o'clock in the morning after 12–14 hours of nightly
05 fasting because these values are affected by basic circadian
06 rhythms.
07   The laboratory test values are given in an older system of
08 units and in the international system of units (SI-units).
09   Despite these precautions, please be aware that the range
10 of normal laboratory values in your country may differ from
11 the values in the tables presented here. Please refer also to
12 the designation of normal values as given by your laboratory.

Blood System – 1481521

Table 1

Peripheral Blood – 4181521

Determination	Restorative Sequence	Units	SI-Units
1	2	3	4
Hemoglobin	4218543		
male	81432142	13–17.5 g/dL	130–175 g/L (2.02–2.71 mmol/L)
female	2154321	12–16 g/dL	120–160 g/L (1.86–2.48 mmol/L)
Erythrocytes	518432129		
male	81543212	4.0–5.6 M in 1 µL	4×10^{12}–5.6×10^{12}/L
female	2143215	3.4–5.0 M in 1 µL	3.4×10^{12}–5.0×10^{12}/L
Color index	81432152	0.86–1.1	0.86–1.1
Leukocytes[1]	514854240		
male	514852187	4,300–11,300 in 1 µL	4.3×10^{9}–11.3×10^{9}/L
female	8231454	3,200–10,200 in 1 µL	3.2×10^{9}–10.2×10^{9}/L

[1] The number of leukocytes varies in the course of 24 hours (maximum in the evening hours); an increase can be observed by muscular activity, emotional stress, intake of protein rich foods and a drastic change in the surrounding temperature.

Determination	Restorative Sequence	Units	SI-Units
Platelet Count in 1 µL Blut[2]	5148154	180000 -320000[2]	180x10⁹ -320x10⁹/l
Retikulozyten	518231418	2 -12 %	0,5 -1,2 %
ESR (Erythrocyte Sedimentation Rate)[3]	514832101		
male	514254351	1 -14 mm/h	
female	4218321	2 -20 mm/h	
Hematocrit – HCT (percentage of blood comprised of red blood cells)	148542118		
male	5421852	40 -54 %	
female	4321852	36 -42 %	

[2] Stimulation of the sympathetic-adrenal system and physical exercise influence the values.
[3] Elevated values in healthy people during pregnancy, after vaccination, dry food nutrition and fasting.

Table 2

Differential Leukocyte Count (WBC Differential Count) – 1489121

Cell Type	Restorative Sequence	%	Number of cells in Thousands per mL Blood	SI-Units
Myelocytes	1842142	0	0	
Metamyelocytes	1844152	0	0	
Neutrophils (granulocytes):	485148293			
banded	514832102	1–6	40–300	0.04– 0,3 x 10⁹/L
segmented	518432128	47–72	2,000–5,500	2–5.5 x 10⁹/L
Eosinophils[1] (granulocytes)	5482151	0,5–5	20–300	0.02–0.3 x 10⁹/L
Basophils (granulocytes)	518432120	0–1	0–65	0–0.065 x 10⁹/L
Lymphocytes	8514321	19–37	1,200–3,000	1.2–3 x 10⁹/L
Monocytes	514232191	3–11	90–600	0.09–0.6 x 10⁹/L

[1] Minimum value: mornings, Maximum value: at night.

Erythrocytes – 518432127

Erythrocytes	Restorative Sequence	Units	SI-Units
1	2	3	4
Osmotic resistance of erythrocytes:	148542145		
minimum	18543210	0.48–0.46%	
maximum	58432142	0.34–0.32%	
Fresh blood, average	5184321	0.20–0.40%	
Incubated blood, average	518543299	0.20–0.65%	
MCV (mean corpuscular volume)	5184514	76–96 µm³	76–96 fL[1]

1	2	3	4
MCH (mean corpuscular hemoglobin)	5854321	27–33	0.42–0.52 fmol/L
MCHC (mean corpuscular Hb concentration)	8543154	30–38%	4.65–5.89 µmol/ erythrocyte
Erythrocyte diameter	5142185	5–6.9 µm (12.5% of the erythrocytes)	
		7–8 µm (75% of the erythrocytes)	
		8.1–9 µm (12.5% of the erythrocytes)	

[1] fl – Femtoliter (10^{15} l)

Morphology of the Blood Platelets (Thrombocytogram) – 1845481

Thrombocyte types – for restoration in cases of pathological values.

Thrombocytes:	young – 18543213	4%
	mature – 4854514	81%
	old – 514858451	5%
	irritated – 4851451	3%
	degenerative form – 514853258	2%
	with vacuolization – 514231481	5%

Table 3

Cytology, Bone Marrow Aspirate (Sternum) – 1848432
Cell Types - 514321541

Cell Type	Restorative Sequence	Normal Range in %
1	2	3
Undifferentiated blast cell	1845421	0.1–1.1
Myeloblast	4851321	0.2–1.7
Neutrophil:	5142184	
Promyelocytes	514254355	1.0–4.1
Myelocytes	518432125	7.0–12.2
Metamyelocytes	5182321	8.0–15.0
banded	514231482	12.8–23.7
segmented	514832103	13.1–24.1
All neutrophils	5145321	52.7–68.9

1	2	3
Basophils all generations	9998143	0 - 0,5
All Erythrokaryocytes	1894321	14,5 - 26,5
Erythroblasts	1487121	0.2 - 1,1
Pronormoblasts (Pronormocytes)	518432123	0,1 - 1,2
Normoblasts (Normocytes)	518432124	
basophil	548432125	1,4 - 4,6
polychromatophilic	514832108	8,9 - 16,9
orthochromatic	518432122	0,8 - 5,6
Monocytes	5484314	0,7 - 3,1
Lymphocytes	1485321	4,3 - 13,7
Plasma cells	518432134	0,1 - 1,8
Reticular cells	518432137	0,1 - 1,6
Megakaryocytes	514832107	0 - 0,6
Myelokaryocytes (1000 per 1 μL)	5143121	41,6 - 195,2
Megakaryocytes (1000 per 1 μL)	5999911	20 - 100
Leuko-erythroblastic ratio	148542199	2,1 - 4,5
Maturation:	5482132	
Erythrokaryocytes	548451238	0,7 - 0,9
Neutrophil	514832105	0,5 - 0,9

Table 4

Morphological Cytology, Lymph Node,
Calculation per 1000 Cells – 1891821

Cell Type	Restorative Sequence	Normal Range %
Lymphoblasts	5148213	0,1 – 0,9
Prolymphocytes	518432135	5,3 – 16,4
Lymphocytes	5421532	67,8 – 90,0
Reticular cells	5182134	0 – 2,6
Plasma cells	5482142	0 – 5,3
Monocytes	548432188	0,2 – 5,8
Mast cells	543218823	0 – 0,5
Neutrophil granulocytes	5145421	0 – 0,5
Eosinophil granulocytes	5488121	0 – 0,3
Basophil granulocytes	5821452	0 – 0,2

Table 5

Morphological Cytology, Spleen, Calculation per 1000 Cells – 1899145

Cell Type	Restorative Sequence	Normal Range %
Lymphoblasts	1854548	0 – 0,2
Prolymphocytes	5842214	1 – 10,5
Lymphocytes	8542145	57 – 84,5
Reticular cells	9999991	0,5 – 1,8
Plasma cells	8887777	0 – 0,3
Erythrokaryocytes	8914214	0 – 0,2
Myelocytes	514832191	0 – 0,4
Metamyelocytes	584321591	0 – 0,1
Neutrophil granulocytes	548132174	1,0 – 7,0
Eosinophil granulocytes	5485142	0,2 – 1,5
Basophil granulocytes	3214852	0,1 – 1,0

Table 6

Coagulation and Fibrinolytic Activity of the Blood – 751483218

Determination	Restorative Sequence	Units
1	2	3
Coagulation time	51432141	
venous	5851321	5 - 10 min
capillary	3148514	Begin 30 sec–2 min, end 3–5 min
Bleeding time	51454328	Not more than 4 min
Thromboelastography (TEG)	514832193	
Reaction time (R)	548543234	5–7 min
Clot formation time (K)	5158321	3–5 min
Maximum amplitude (MA)	5483248	45–55 mm
Plasma recalcification time	51485432	60–120 sec
Tolerance of citrated plasma to Heparin	5488312	10–16 min
in 75% of patients [1]		10–14 min
in 90% of patients [1]		10–16 min
Tolerance of oxalated plasma to Heparin	5488345	7–15 min
Tolerance of plasma to Protamine sulfate	5488314	7–9 sec

[1] According to various authors.
[2] In parentheses: SI-Units

1	2	3
Prothrombin time (PT) using plasma	5488415	Index 90–105% or 12–20 sec
Prothrombin time capillary blood	514231499	Index 93–107%
Antithrombin activity	514852191	90–110%
Prothrombin consumption	8542314	80–100%
Fibrinolytic activity plasma	3148542	3–4 hrs
Plasma fibrinogen – Factor 1 (weight method)	4851321	200–400 mg% (2–4 g/L) [2]
Plasma fibrinogen – Factor 1 (calorimetric method)	514832192	250–300 mg% (2.5–3 g/L) [2]
Plasma fibrinogen (Ruthberg's method)	5145142	8–13 mg/mL (8–13 g/L) [2]
Plasma fibrinogen B test	14814325	Not determined
Factor XIII (fibrin stabilizing factor)	485142175	40–50 U
Thromboplastin generation test (Plasma, Thrombocytes, Serum)	514832194	7–12 sec
Factor II (Prothrombin)	4854451	85–110%
Factor V (accelerator globulin)	548132132	85–110%
Factor VIII (proconvertin)	54321483	80–100%
Factor X Concentration	45481451	60–130%
Factor VII	5485145	65–135%
Fibrin split products	1483214	Negative reaction
Partial Thromboplastin time (activated)	4518231	35–50 s
Plasma soluble fibrin monomer complex	518432132	0.35–0.47 U
Platelet adhesion assay	5481253	25–55%
Aggregation time stimulation by ADF	1483545	75–195%
Platelet disaggregation time	5483212	45–175 sec

Table 7

ABO System Forward Typing with Serum
(containing antibodies) – 148542117 [1]

Blood Type	Restorative Sequence [2]	Reaction Result using Standardized Serum			
1	2	3	4	5	6
		0αß (1)	Aß (II)	Bα(III)	AB(IV)
0(1) [3]	148542188	-	-	-	-
A(II)	145432171	+	-	+	-
B(III)	1454213	+	+	-	-
AB(IV)	4444888	+	+	+	-

[1] This Restorative Sequence restores all blood types. [2] These Restorative Sequences restore the respective blood type. [3] Russian blood type designation in parentheses.

Table 8

ABO System Back Typing (patient's blood serum is mixed with standard Erythrocytes) – 1834567

Blood Serum	Restorative Sequence	Reaction Result using Standardized Erythrocytes		
		0(I)	A(II)	B(III)
0αß (I)	148542185	-	+	+
Aß (II)	145432182	-	-	+
Bα (III)	1454213	-	+	-
AB (IV)	4444888	-	-	-

URINE – 1852155

Physical Characteristics – 85432181

Determination	Restorative Sequence	Results
Urine volume/d	1821452	800 – 1500 ml [1]
Relative density of morning sample	1824351	1020 – 1026 [2]
Maximal osmotic concentration	5432152	910 mosm/l
Color	5143212	Straw-colored
Transparency	3814321	Transparent

[1] Polyuria physiologically increases the desire for fluids and triggers neurogenic factors.
[2] The value fluxuates greatly in the course of 24 hrs.

Table 9

Chemical Constituents of Urine – 1485218

Determination	Restorative Sequence	Units	SI-Units
1	2	3	4
pH Reaction	51432181	Neutral or slightly acid [1]	
Protein	54321858	absent, traces (25–70 mg/d) [2]	0.025–0.070 g/d

[1] An alkaline reaction appears with a vegetable diet, alkaline drinks and at the height of digestion.
[2] Transitory proteinuria appears as a result of muscular activity or physical strain.

1	2	3	4
Sugar	5432841	absent, traces (not more than 0.02%) [3]	
Acetone	543218848	absent	
Keton bodies	5185411	absent	
Urobilin bodies	5148218	absent	
Bilirubin	5145821	absent [4]	
Ammonia	5421321	0.6–1.3 g/d	36–78 mmol/d
Uric acid	518888842	270–600 mg/d	1.62–3.6 mmol/d
Purin bases:	9999991		
Hypoxanthin	1998214	9.7 mg/d	
Xanthin	5148211	6.1 mg/d	
Urea	5814321	20–35 g/d	333.0–582.8 mmol/d
Creatinine:	5854321	0.5–2 g/d	4.4–17.6 mmol/d
male	814254351	1–2 g/d	8.8–17.6 mmol/d
female	5182843	0.5–1.6 g/d	4.4–14.08 mmol/d
Creatine	518432139	absent	
Alpha-amylase	5821341	20–160 mg starch (h/mL)	20–160 g (h/L)
Uropepsin	518432179	38–96 mg/d	
Potassium	5142311	1.5–3 g/d	38.4–76.7 mmol/d
Sodium	5148211	3–6 g/d	130.5–261.0 mmol/d
Chlorine	5148544	120–170 mE/L (600–740 mg%)	120–170 mmol/L
Inorganic phosphorus	5184322	0.6–1.2 g/d	0.019–0.038 mmol/d

[3] Functional Glucosuria appears with emotional stress, over-abundance of sugar in nutrients and increase of adrenalin. [4] Intake of Antipyrine yields a false positive reaction.

Urine Sediment – 5148211

	Restorative Sequence	Results
Epithelial cells	8148211	0–3 in field of vision
Leukocytes	5188911	
male	5191522	0–2 in field of vision
female	543218845	1–2 in field of vision
Erythrocytes	8910101	mimimal
Casts	5148514	none
Mucus	5148512	none
Bacteria	514831254	not more than 50,000 in 1 mL
Inorganic sediment	514218878	
Acid reaction	8432111	Uric acid, Urate, Calcium oxalate
Alkaline reaction	2222543	amorphous phosphates, ammonium biurates, tripolyphosphate

Urine Analysis		Restorative Sequence	Results
Kakowski-Addis Method		514218897	
In 24 hr urine collection:			
	Leukocytes	1234588	up to 2,000,000 (2x10⁶/d)
	Erythrocytes	5488511	up to 1,000,000 (1x10⁶/d)
	Casts	514548823	up to 20,000 (2x10⁴/d)
Nechiporenko Method:		148851481	
In 1 mL urine:			
	Leukocytes	5488144	up to 4 000
	Erythrocytes	514548891	up to 1 000
	Casts	1888455	0–1 per 4 U
Sternheimer–Malbin Method		1454588	
Active Leukocytes in 1 mL urine		1454588	from 1 to 200

Table 10

Kidney Function Tests – 1485454

Type of Test	Restorative Sequence	Method	Results
Dilution test	1454818	according to Volhard after drinking 1.5 L water	More than 50% of the consumed liquid is eliminated after 2 hrs; the rest after 3–4 hrs. The density sinks to 1001–1003. Urine amount in portions of 50–500 mL.
Concentration test	1451855	according to Volhard	Urine amount in portions of 50–60 mL, density after 4–8 hrs reaches 1028–1035.
Simnitzki test	1458815		Daily diuresis yields 2/3–3/4 of the amount consumed in 24 hrs. Density: 1004¬1024.
Rebberg's method	1458817	Creatinine clearance in blood und urine	Glomerular filtration 75–125 mg/min. Reabsorption 98.2–98.8%
Indigo-carmine test	5454888	intravenous application of 20 mL 0.4% indigo-carmine	Elimination of dyed urine after 5 –10 min.
Volume of the tubular secretion	5884555	application of Phenol red	Elimination with urine: after 15 min at least 25% of the dye used.

Intestinal Contents - 1485458

Determination	Restorative Sequence	Results
Total amount in 24 hrs	1823454	100–250 g
Consistency	148543287	fairly firm
Form	148543290	cylindrical
Color	512314542	brown
PH Reaction	5485451	neutral or slightly alkaline
Mucus, blood	518432181	none

Stool Microscopy – 1854532

Determination	Restorative Sequence	Results
Muscle fibers	5421321	none or digested ones that lost transverse markings
Cell tissue	518432183	none or few fibers
Fats	518432187	none or small amounts
Fatty acids, fatty soaps	145432191	small amounts
Vegetable fiber	518432189	
digested	5182321	few cells or cell groups
undigested	5148345	varied amounts
Starch	5821314	none
Detritus	5142389	varied amounts
Mucus, Epithelial cells	8432548	none
Leukocytes	82143213	few

Chemical Constituents of the Intestinal Contents – 5145814
(Calculated to 24-hr amounts)

Determination	Restorative Sequence	Results
1	2	3
Nitrogen	1248510	0.25–2 g
Protein	0100101	none
Bilirubin	1484545	none
Water	1489891	48–200 mL
Fats	548214583	2.5–10 g.
Potassium	7148565	7–12 mEv
Calcium	6414854	400–900 mg
Coproporphyrin	6651049	200–300 µg
Sodium	5432182	1–5 mEv
Urobilin	148542183	40–280 mg

SALIVA – 514821441

Determination	Restorative Sequence	Results
Amount	18754321	1000–1500 mL/d
Relative density	5843210	1002–1008
pH	14542108	6.0–7.9

Table 11

Chemical Constituents of Saliva – 14542101

Constituent	Restorative Sequence	Content in mg	SI-Units
Nitrogen (non-protein)	1482314	13.0 (37% nitrogen blood)	9.28 mmol/L
Ammonia	5891420	2.0–10.0	1.2–6 μmol/L
Protein	54854321	200.0–400.0	0.2–0.4 g/L
Total calcium	5451231	4.0–8.0	1–2 mmol/L
Carbonates (CO2)	5142843	20–45 mL/100 mL	
Uric acid	5421314	1.5 (40% uric acid in blood)	0.088 mmol/L
Urea	54815425	11.0 (76% urea in blood)	1.83 mmol/L
Potassium	9981521	19–23 mE/L	19–23 mmol/L
Phosphates	5148512	0.005–0.2	0.0016–0.064 mmol/L
Inorganic Phosphorus	5458212	10.0–25.0	3.2–8.08 mmol/L
Chloride	514852193	30.0–60.0	8.46–16.9 mmol/L
Cholesterol	5821542	2.5–9.0	0.065–0.233 mmol/L

Gastric Juice – 5148210

Determination	Restorative Sequence	Results
Amount	5482142	2–3 L/24 hrs
Relative density	5210840	1005
pH	1234542	1.6–1.8

Table 12

Chemical Constituents of the Gastric Juice – 8912014

Constituent	Restorative Sequence	Units	SI-Units
Non-protein nitrogen	814854218	20–48 mg%	14.3–34.4 mmol/L
Urea and ammonia	548214891	7–14 mg%	4.99–9.99 mmol/L
Amino acids	5124312	2–8 mg/L	1.43–5.7 mmol/L
Chloride	5812543	550 mg%	155.1 mmol/L
Free Hydrogen chloride	1584321	200 mg%	20 mmol/L
Uric acid	514832198	0.8–2 mg%	47.6–118.9 µmol/L
Potassium	4821358	21.8–137.7 mg%	5.6–35.3 mE/L (mmol/L)
Sodium	4812844	72–435.4 mg%	31.3–189.3 mE/L (mmol/L)

Gastric Juice (Empty Stomach) – 48142123

Determination	Restorative Sequence	Results
Amount	514854148	5–40 mL
General acid content	9998111	not more than 20–30 titration units
Free Hydrochloric acid	518432191	up to 15 titration units
Pepsin	5842144	0–21 mg%
Basal acid output:	8142521	
Gastric juice specimens are collected In a fasted state in intervals of 15 min	81454322	50–100 mL
Acid output	5424321	40–460 titration units; 40–60 mE/L (mmol/L)[1]
Free Hydrochloric acid	5142811	20–40 titration units;
20–40 mE/L (mmol/L)[1]	5142811	20 - 40 Titrationseinheiten; 20 - 40 mäqv/l(mmol/l) [1]
Hydrochloric acid, hourly	514254481	50–150mg; 1.5–5.5 Me/L (mmol/L)[1]
Free Hydrochloric acid, hourly	54321482	1–4 mE/L
Pepsin, hourly	1234567	10–40 mg

[1] SI-Einheiten.

Stimulants of Gastric Secretion – 12345717

Determination	Restorative Sequence	Results
Parenteral administration of stimulants:	1451891	
Histamine dichloride SC	1248512	0.008 mg/kg
Histamine phosphate	1248542	0.01 mg/kg

Secretion occurs after 7–10 min, maximum after 45–60 min; last 1–1.5 hrs, decreases gradually.
Maximum stimulation according to Key:
    Histamine dichloride: 0.024 mg/kg – 1248542
    Histamine phosphate: 0.04 mg/kg – 1248542
    Apply Antihistamines (2 mL of 2% dilution of Suprastin) 30 min before the administration of Histamine
    Insulin (12 units SC, 0.15 – 0.20 units/kg body weight IV

Enteric stimulants:
    200 mL 7–10% broth of dried cabbage (according to Petrowa and Riss, unified)
    0.2 g Coffein in 400 mL water (according to Katsch and Kalk)
    300 mL meat broth, cooked from 300 g meat in 1 L water (according to Simnitzki)
    200 mL cabbage juice (according to Leporski)
    15 mL 96% ethanol in 285 mL water (according to Ermann)

Table 13

Stimulated Gastric Secretion – 148542173

Determination	Restorative Sequence	Stimulant	
		Cabbage juice, broth	Histamine
Volume of gastric juice per hr/mL	1111211	50–110	100-150
Acid output	1485412	40–60	80-100
Free Hydrogen chloride	148542177	20–40	65-85
Titration units:			
Hydrochloric acid, hourly, mE/L	1851421	1.5–6	8-14
Free Hydrochloric acid, hourly, mE/L	1848521	1.0–4.5	6,5-12
Pepsin, hourly, mg	1821512	20–40	50-90

Microscopy of the Stomach Contents – 1891512

Determination	Restorative Sequence	Result
1	2	3
Starchy granules	1894512	determinable
Muscle fibers	1111110	none

© Г. П. Грабовой, 1999

1	2	3
Fat	0124895	none
Plant cells	5814321	none
Epithel	548543281	small amount
Erythrocytes	514854251	none
Leukocytes	518432199	small amount, deformed
Yeast	514854258	sparse
Sarcine	5145182	none
Lactobacillus	518432197	none

BILE – 514852188
24-Hour Amount 500–1000 mL – 8219931

Table 14

Composition of Bile (g/L) – 1548212

Determination	Restorative Sequence	Hepatic Bile	Bile of the Gall Bladder
Nitrogen	8145214	0.8	4.9
Choline	518432198	0.4–0.9	5.5
Bile acid	1454815	7–14	115
Lecithin	5121314	1.0–5.8	35
Cholesterol	5148212	0.8–2.1	4.3
Protein	514821447	1.4–2.7	4.5
Bilirubin	5182514	0.3–0.6	1.4
α-Amylase	1454521	6–16 g starch (mL•H)	1.67–4.45 mg (L•h)
Trypsin	514854261	50–500 μmol (mL•min)	

Evaluation of Duodenal Contents – 215184321

One Specimen	Restorative Sequence	Result
Amount	1245212	20–35 mL (10 mL in 10 min.)
Color	5124321	golden yellow
Transparency	5124512	transparent
Relative density	1891701	1007–1015
pH reaction	5172456	slightly alkaline

Table 15

Bile Acid Stimulation – 1284521

Determination	Restorative Sequence	Bile	Bile
		in the gall bladder	in the bile ducts
Amount	1285514	20–50 mL	30 mL
Color	5124851	dark brown (olive colored)	golden yellow
Transparency	1821532	clear	clear
Relative density	89143214	1016–1032	1007–1010
pH Reaction	8432151	alkaline	alkaline
Bilirubin	5124814	15–45 mg%	18 mg%
		(SI: 256.5–769.7 µmol/L)	(SI: 307.8 µmol/L)

Table 16

Microscopic Examination of the Bile Specimens – 1485451

Determination	Restorative Sequence	Portion		
		I	II	III
Epithel	5184512	a few	sparse	
Leukocytes in the visual field	235184321	2–4	5–10	2–4
Mucus	148542175	in varying amounts		
Cholesterol and Calcium bilirubinate crystals	1485142	–	sparse	–

Table 17

Cerebrospinal Fluid – 1489100

Determination	Restorative Sequence	Units	SI-Units
1	2	3	4
Amount	1891421	100–150 mL	
Relative density	5451422	1006–1008	

1	2	3	4
Pressure, lying	52143213	150–200 mm Hg	
Pressure, sitting	5214321	300–400 mm Hg	
Color	1222227	colorless, seldom yellow, grayish	
Cytosis (increased cell count) in 1 µL:	1845451		
Ventricular fluid	5814212	0–1	
Cisternal fluid	5814321	0–1	
Lumbar fluid	5812432	2–3	
pH	514821453	7.35–7.80	
Protein (total)	775184321	15–45 mg%	0.15–0.45 g/L
Lumbar fluid	5148512	22–33 mg%	0.22–0.33 g/L
Cisternal fluid	5821531	10–22 mg%	0.10–0.22 g/L
Ventricular fluid	5482999	12–20 mg%	0.12–0.20 g/L
Glucose	5891488	50–70 mg%	2.78–3.89 mmol/L
Chloride ions	8142835	425–460 mg%	120–130 mE/L mmol/L

Biochemistry of the Blood – 514832189

Table 18

Protein and Protein Fractions – 185843218

Determination	Restorative Sequence	Units	SI-Units
Protein (total) blood serum	1814542	6.5–8.5 g%	65–68 g/L
Albumin	815184321	4–5 g%	40–50 g/L
Globulin	5182321	2–3 g%	20–30 g/L
Fibrinogen	58432149	0.2–0.4 g%	2–4 g/L

Table 19

Protein Fractions[1] (Paper Electrophoresis) – 148542138

Determination	Restorative Sequence	A. A. Pokrovski (1969), relative %	F. I. Komarov and others (1982), relative %	W. G. Kolb and others (1976) (n=100)		
				relative %	g%	SI: -g/L
Albumin	4821512	56,6 - 66,8	51 - 61,5	61,5 ± 0,7	4,97 ± 0,07	49,7 ± 0,7
Globulin:	5814321					
α_1	5121451	3 - 5,6	3,6 - 5,6	5,5 ± 0,21	0,45 ± 0,02	4,5 ± 0,2
α_2	8910104	6,9 - 10,5	5,1 - 8,3	6,7 ± 0,20	0,56 ± 0,02	5,6 ± 0,2
ß	1482182	7,3 - 12,5	9 - 13	9,2 ± 0,24	0,76 ± 0,02	7,6 ± 0,2
y	1424214	12,8 - 19	15 - 22	16,8 ± 0,34	1,39 ± 0,03	13,9 ± 0,3

[1] The blood contains 100 different protein components. Using paper electrophoresis, the protein is separated into 5 fractions, with agarose gel 7 – 8, with starch gel 16 –18, with immunoelectrophoresis into approximately 30 fractions.

Tests for Dysproteinemia – 1421514

Test	Restorative Sequence	Description
Weltmann reaction	1821521	0.4–0.5 mL CaCl2 solution (5–7 test tubes)
Mercuric chloride (Sulema) reaction	1421542	1.6–2.2 mL Mercury dichloride
Thymol turbidity test	5148512	0–4 Units

Table 20

Rest Nitrogen and its Components – 91854321

Determination	Restorative Sequence	Content		Nitrogen in % of the total remaining Nitrogen
		mg%	SI-Units	
		Blood Serum		
1	2	3	4	5
Rest Nitrogen	5148212	20–40	7.06–14.1 mmol/L	100
Urea	5432180	20–40	3.3–6.6 mmol/L	50 (46 – 60)

1	2	3	4	5
Amino acid nitrogen	148542161	2.0–4.3	1.43–3.07 mmol/L	25
Uric acid	815518432	2–6.4	0.12–0.38 mmol/L	4
Creatine:	885184321			
male	295184321	0.2–0.7	13–53 µmol/L	5
female	5432148	0.4–0.9	27–71 µmol/L	2.5
Creatinine:	5148211			
male	5184321	1–2	0.088–0.177mmol/L	
female	5182144	0.5–1.6	0.044–0.141 mmol/L	
Ammonia	489152141	0.03–0.06	21.4–42.8	
Remaining non-protein substances	1482155			13
Polypeptides, Nucleotides and others	5148514			
Xanthoproteic reaction	54321488	20 U		
Creatine, blood	5148215	3–4 mg%	229–305 µmol/L	
Creatine, plasma	1485425	1–1.5mg%	76.3–114.5 µmol/L	
Blood urea nitrogen (BUN)	5142182	9–14 mg%	3.18–4.94 mmol/L	

Table 21

Amino Acids Blood Plasma – 1824542

Amino Acids	Restorative Sequence	Proportion		Amino Acids	Proportion	
		mg%	µmol/L		mg%	µmol/L
Glycine (Glycocoll)	5121542	2,8 - 3,0		Arginin	1,6 - 3,0	91,8 - 172,2
Alanine	5482142	3,2 - 5,6	359,0 - 628,3	Lysin	2,1 - 5,3	143,9 - 363,1
Methionine	5481214	0,3 - 0,5	20,1 - 33,6	Glutaminsäure	0,8 - 1,1	54,4 - 74,8
Valine	518254442	2,2 - 3,2	188,1 - 273,6	Glutamin	7,5 - 8,3	513,8 - 568,6
Leucine	5185148	1,7 - 3,3	129,7 - 251,8	Prolin	2,6	222,2
Isoleucine	5152142	1,6 - 2,0	121,1 - 152,6	Serin	1,16	110,4
Tyrosine	5482142	1,4 - 1,5	77,3 - 82,8	Treonin	1,9 - 2,1	159,6 - 176,4
Phenylalanine	1854212	1,4 - 1,9	84,7 - 114,9	Histidin	1,7 - 2,1	109,7 - 135,5
Tryptophan	1854511	1,0	49,0	Zystein	2,0 - 3,0	166,6 - 249,9

Table 22

Lipids in Blood Plasma – 1845489

Blood Lipid Fractions	Restorative Sequence	Result	
		Units	SI-Units
Lipids [1]	1454525	350 - 800mg%	4,6 - 10,4 mmol/l
Phospholipids	5154812	150 - 380 mg%	1,95 - 4,9 mmol/l
Lipoid phosphorus	1852312	6,1 - 14,5 mg%	1,97 - 4,68 mmol/l
Neutral fats	1485214	0 - 200 mg%	
Triglycerides (blood serum) [1]	18543215	50 - 150 mg%	0,565 - 1,695 mmol/l
Non-esterified fatty acid	145454577	20 - 50 mg%	0,71 - 1,75 mmol/l
Free fatty acid	8912542	0,3 - 0,8 mäq/l	0,3 - 0,8 μmol/l
Total cholesterol [2]	1482121	120 -250 mg%	3,11 - 6,48 mmol/l
Free cholesterol	1482541	40 - 90 mg% (30 - 40% d.ges.)	1,04 - 2,33 mmol/l
Esterified cholesterol	1248542	90 - 135 mg% (60 - 70% d.ges.)	2,33 - 3,49 mmol/l
α-High-density Lipoprotein (HDL) α-Lipoprotein (25 – 30%)	1454214	220 mg%	2,2 g/l
male	5482142	125 -4 25 mg%	1,25 - 4,25 g/l
female	542143221	250-650 mg%	2,5 - 6,5 g/l
Low-density Lipoprotein (LDL) ß-Lipoprotein (65 – 75%)	174845421	350 - 450 mg%	3 - 4,5 g/l
		35–55 IU optical density (turbidimetric method)	

[1] Test only on empty stomach.
[2] The value is differs with age.

Table 23

Total Cholesterol in Relation to Age – 1482152

Age in Years	Restorative Sequence	Result (Keys and others, 1950)		Age in Years	Result (Friedrichsen and others, 1967)	
		mg%	mmol/L		mg%	mmol/L
1	2	3	4	5	6	7
20	1482142	101–189	2.6–4.9	0–19	120–230	3.1–5.9
30	1821251	108–218	2.8–5.7	21–29	120–240	3.1–6.2

1	2	3	4	5	6	7
40	543218891	128–237	3.3–6.2	30–39	140–270	3.6–7.02
50	1489100	145–270	3.8–7.02	40–49	150–310	3.9–8.06
60	0018914	165–258	4.3–6.7	50–59	160–330	4.2–8.9
70	0010101	129–246	3.4–6.4			

Table 24

Lipoproteids in the Blood Serum – 1482142

Determination	Restorative Sequence	Lipoprotein Types			Chylo-microns
		HDL (LPBP)	LDL (LPNP)	VLDL (LPONP)	
Relative density	5481214	1063 - 1210	1010 - 1063	1010 - 930	930
Molecular mass	5182142	180 - 380 tausend	2 200 000	3 - 128 Mio	-
Total serum protein (%)	5182414	50 - 57	21 - 2 2	5 - 12	2
Lipids (%)	5482121	43 - 50	78 - 79	88 - 95	98
Free cholesterol (%)	5121489	2 - 3	8 - 10	3 - 5	2
Esterified cholesterol	1842514	19 - 29	36 - 37	10 - 13	4 - 5
Phosphor lipids (%)	514854272	22 - 24	20 - 22	13 - 20	4 - 7
Cholesterol (total)	51245422				
Phosphor lipids, %	5148542	1,0	2,3	0,9	1,1
Triglyceride, %	5148212	4 - 8	11 - 12	50 - 60	84 - 87

Table 25

Carbohydrate Metabolism of the Blood – 514214891

Determination	Restorative Sequence	Units	SI-Units
1	2	3	4
Glycogen	785184321	12–21 mg%	
Glucose	1485451		
Hagedorn-Jensen method [1]			

[1] This method is non-specific; in addition to the Glucose, these reducing non-sugars are determined: glutathione, creatinine, uric acid, ascorbic acid, glucuronic acid, etc.

1	2	3	4
Whole blood	1234681	80–120 mg%, of which:	4.44–6.66 mmol/L
		15–30% are reducing substances	
		55–90 mg% is Glucose	3.05–5.27 mmol/L
O-Toluidine method [2]:	148542163		
Whole blood	1485418	60–100 mg%	3.33–5.55 mmol/L
Plasma	548214547	60–110 mg%	3.33–6.1 mmol/L
Glucose oxidase method [3]:	5451481	56–94 mg%	
Glucose in whole blood	5184512	56–94 mg%	3.10–5.21 mmol/L
Glucose in plasma and serum	5148512	55–100 mg%	3.05–5.55 mmol/L
Fructose	5182142	0.1–0.5 mg%	0.56–2.77 mmol/L
Galactose, serum	1821421	2–17 mg%	0.11–0.94 mmol/L
Lactic acid	5421431	9–16 mg%	0.99–1.78 mmol/L
Pyruvic acid	5481214	0.4–0.8 mg%	45.6–91.2 μmol/L
Acetone	5142182	none	
Oxaloacetic acid	1821451	2.5–6 mg%	0.43–1.033 mmol/L

[2] The O-Toluidine method is not specific for glucose, because galactine, xylose, dextran, hoxose, pantose disaccharides and glucuronic acid may also react with o-toluidine. The value produced by this test exaggerates the content of hemoglobin, bilirubin and protein in the blood.
[3] A highly specific method, but ascorbic acid and antibiotics of the tetracycline type must not be taken 3 days prior.

Table 26

Glycoprotein and Its Components – 5148512

Determination	Restorative Sequence	Units	SI-Units
Glycoprotein	5184542	120–160 mg%	1.2–1.6 g/L
Protein-bound Hexose	1482154	105–115 mg%	1.05–1.65 g/L
Seromucoids:	5121481		
Hexose	1425128	22–28 mg%	0.22–0.28 g/L
Turbidimetric method	4812523	0.13–0.20 IU optical density	
Sialic acid	5142821	135–200 units, 62–73 mg% N-Acetylneuraminic acid	2.0–3.36 mmol/L
Bilirubin Metabolism in Blood – 548132177			
Total bilirubin	5414218	0.65 (0.5–1.2) mg%	11.12 (8.6–20.5) μmol/L
Conjugated bilirubin (BC)	5128143	0.15 mg%	2.57 μmol/L
Unconjugated bilirubin (BU)	52143218	0.50 mg% (75% of total)	8.6 μmol/Ll

Table 27

Electrolytes and Trace Minerals in the Blood – 518431181

Determination	Restorative Sequence	Units	SI-Units
Calcium, serum	1485321	9–12 mg% (4.5–6 mE/L)	2.25–3.0 mmol/L
Magnesium, serum	514831298	1.7–2.4 mg% (1.5–2.0 mE/L)	0.70–0.99 mmol/L
Chloride, serum	1482182	340–390 mg% (95–110 mE/L)	95.9–109.9 mmol/L
Phosphorus (inorganic)	1482152	2–4 mg% (1.2–2.3 mE/L)	0.65–1.30 mmol/L
Iron, serum	1481521	70–170 µg%	12.5–30.4 mol/L
Transferrin, free	18543216	0.150–0.230 mg%	0.0015–0.0023 g/L
Transferrin, total	1821542	0.300–0.400 mg%	0.0030–0.0040 g/L
Copper, serum	1481214	70–140 µg%	11.02–22.04 µmol/L
Ceruloplasmin	1482182	27+-1.44 mg%	0.27+-0.014 g/L
Potassium, plasma	1421542	13.6–20.8 mg% (3.48–5.3 mE/L)	3.48–5.3 mmol/L
Potassium, erythrocytes	5124821	305–374 mg% (77.8–95.7 mE/L)	77.8–95.7 mmol/L
Sodium, plasma	1421542	300–360 mg% (130.5–156.6 mE/L)	130.5–156.6 mmol/L
Sodium, erythrocytes	1482121	31–50 mg% (13.48–21.75 mE/L)	13.k48–21.75 mmol/L
Lithium	514821458	0.35–1.4 mg% (0.5–2 mE/L)	0.5–2.0 µmol/L

Table 28

Blood pH – 1454821

Determination	Restorative Sequence	SI-Units
1	2	3
Concentration of hydrogen ions (pH):	1897012	
male	0014248	7.36–7.42
female	0148000	7.37–7.42

1	2	3
CO_2 partial pressure:	5182421	
male	5128314	35.8–46.6 mmHg
female	2185432	32.5–43.7 mmHg
Buffer base (BB)	514821461	44.9–51.9 mE/L blood
Base excess (BE)	1482185	
male	5148218	2.4–2.3 mE/L blood
female	2100011	3.3–1.2 mE/L blood
Standard bicarbonate (SB)	1845421	18.8–24.0 mE/L plasma
Bicarbonate	555184321	21.3–24.8 mE/L plasma
Total CO2	3148222	21–26 mE/L plasma

Blood Enzymes – 1482542

Determination	Restorative Sequence	Units	SI-Units
1	2	3	4
Amylase	148542114	12–32 mg starch (mg/h)	12–32 g/(h*L)
Aspartate transaminase (SGOT)	148582114	8–40 U	0.1–0.45 mmol/(h*L)
Alanine transaminase (ALT)	1824821	5–30 U	0.1–0.68 mmol/(h*L)
Lactate dehydrogenase (total)	1482542	0.8–4.0 μm pyruvate (mL/h)	0.8–4.0 mmol/(h*L)
Lactate dehydrogenase (urea-stable)	5481212	25–36% of total	
Cholinesterase	1821541	160–340 μm acetic acid (mL*h)	160–340 mmol/(h*L)
y-Glutamyl transpeptidase (GGT)	1482542		0.6–3.96 mmol/(h*L)
Lipase	5821321	0.28 ME/L	
Alkaline Phosphatase (ALP) (total)	1481212	1–3 μmol para-nitrophenol (mL*h)	1.0–3.0 mmol/(h*L)
Alkaline Phosphatase (ALP) (total)		0.5–1.3 μmol inorganic phosphorus (mL*h)	
Isoenzymes	1215421	up to 20% of total	
Acid phosphatase (total)	1248212	0.025–0.12 μmol inorganic	
phosphorus (mL*h)		1–4 mkmol(ml/min)	60-40mkmol(ml´h)
Trypsin	148542187	1–4 μmol(mL/min)	60–240 μmol(mL*h)
Fructose 1-phosphate aldolase	1821512	0–1 U	
Fructose 1.6-biphosphate aldolase	1482543	3–8 U	
Sorbitol dehydrogenase	1421821	0–0.02 μmol/(mL*h)	

1	2	3	4
Glucose-6-phosphate dehydrogenase in Erythrocytes	148542152	negative	
Creatine phosphokinase (CK, CKP)	1851421	10–110 ME	0.60–66 mmol
inorganic phosphorus (h*L)	5148212		
Isoenzyme – CKP:	5148212		
BB	5182411	none	
MB	5843212	4–6% of total	
MM	4821542	94–96% of total	

Immunological Blood Values – 148542153

Determination	Restorative Sequence	Result
Antihyaluronidase	4812153	up to 300 U (AH)
Antistreptolysin O	1454512	250 U
Waaler-Rose test	1482125	Agglutination up to titer 1:20
Lysozyme serum	1821542	8–12 µg/mL
Properdin serum	1821543	20–80 hemolytic U
Serum complement	1854521	20–50 hemolytic [1] U
Rheumatoide factor	1821521	Agglutination up to titer 1:20
α-Fetoprotein	5821432	negative
C-reactive protein	5182421	negative
Leukocyte antibodies	5148123	none
DNA antibodies	1482482	none
Cancer Antigens	481854224	none

[1] The value for females is up to 10% lower than males and is reduced during pregnancy by as much as 30%.

Table 29

Immunoglobulin Content in the Blood Serum – 1481521

	Restorative Sequence	Immunoglobulin Type					
		IgM		IgG		IgA	
		mg%	g/L	mg%	g/L	mg%	g/L
Male	5821451	55–141	0.55–1.41	664–1400	6.64–14.0	103–404	1.03–4.04
Female	3215214	37–195	0.37–1.95	587–1630	5.87–16.3	54–343	0.54–3.43

Table 30

T- and B-Lymphocyte Count in the Blood – 1482123

Cells	Restorative Sequence	%	Absolute Count in 1 μL of Blood
T-Lymphocytes	5814321	74.08+-0.96	1549.58+-69.35
B-Lymphocytes	1458512	21.5+-0.85	432.88+-27.5

Activity Indicators of Neuroendocrine System,[1],[2] – 518432121

Table 31

Pituitary-Adrenal System – 5144831299
Hormone Content in the Blood – 5148212

Hormone	Restorative Sequence	Content in the Blood		Method
		Units	SI-Units	
Adrenocorticotropic hormone (ACTH)	148542191	75–150 pg/mL	16.4–32.8 mmol/L	radio-immuno assay RIA
17-Hydroxycorticosteroids, serum	1482542	10–25 μg/100 mL	280–700 nmol/L	calorimetric
11-Deoxycorticosterone:	1854512			
total [2]	5184999	14–23 μg/100mL	280–700 nmol/L	fluorimetric
free [3]	5199421	5–10% of total		same
Cortisol	5851422	5–23 μg/100mL	140–640 nmol/L	radio-immuno assay
Hydrocortisone	5185142	58+-5.8 ng/mL	160.1+-16 nmol/L	same

[1] The hormone content in blood is lower with progressing age.
[2] The difference in measured values of the same hormone in the blood with the radio-immuno assay as compared to the saturation method is caused by the colligative action of the proteins used.
[3] In pregnancy the value is almost doubled.

Table 32

Content of Hormones and their Metabolites in Urine – 5182321

Hormone	Restorative Sequence	24-hr Specimen		Method
		Units	SI-Units	
17-Ketosteroids:	5148512			
female	5148212	6.4–18.0 mg/d	22.2–62.6 µmol/d	calorimetric
male	9999991	6.6–23.4 mg/d	22.9–81.3 µmol/d	
17-Hydroxycorticosteroids:	1821000			
total	0018542	1.5–7.4 mg/d	4.1–13.7 µmol/d	same
free	4821322	up to 7% of total		
Cortisol (hydrocortisone)	1454542	10–100 µg/d	27.6–276 nmol/d	radio-immuno assay

Table 33

Hypophyseal-Gonadotropic Hormones – 1821454

Hormone	Restorative Sequence	Male	Menstrual Cycle [1]		Pregnancy	Meno-pause
			II	III		
In plasma (RIA)	5148512					
Luteinizing hormone (LH), hormone/mL	514852199	6–23	5–30	75–150	3–40	3–200
Follicle-stimulating hormone (FSH) hormone/mL	5485154	4–25		4–30		4–25
Prolactin (PRL) ng/mL, µg/L	1458215	<20	<23	5–40	<400	
Testosterone ng/100mL	5145421	572		37	114	
Progesterone ng/mL	51421541	0.12–0.30	0.02–0.9	6–30	80–200	
Estrogenes, total ng/mL	52143219	40–115	61–394	122–437	156–350	700–31000
Estriol, total ng/mL	5184214	<2	<2		30–350	<10
Dehydroepiandrosterone (DHEA) ng/mL	1821542	1.7–4.2	2.0	5.2	7.18	0.5–43
In urine	5182132					
Estrogene, total (RIA) µg/s	5214321	5–25	5–25	28–100	22–80	up to 45,000
Dehydroepiandrosterone (DHEA) mg/s	514821465	0–4		0–12	0–4.2	

[1] Menstrual cycle phases: I = Follicular phase, II = Ovulation, III = Luteal phase.

Table 34

Renin-Aldosterone System – 1482152

Determination	Restorative Sequence	Units	SI-Units
Renin activity, plasma:	1482154		
supine position	1821321	1.6+-1.5 µg(l/h)	
upright position	5432151	4.5+-2.9 µg(l/h)	
Aldosterone, plasma:	1482159		
supine position	9149999	3–10 ng/100mL	0.08–0.28 pmol/L
upright position	9114801	5–30 ng/100 mL	0.14–0.83 pmol/L
Aldosterone in Urine (acid-labile conjugate)	1482185	3–15 µg/d	0.083–0.42 nmol/d

Table 35

Thyroid Hormones – 81432157

Determination	Restorative Sequence	Units	SI-Units
Plasma	**4814825**		
Thyroxine, total: adult newborn	5481214	5-10mkg/100ml 11,5-24 µg/100mL	65-129pmol/L 148-310pmol/L
Thyroxine, free	1484545	0.02–0.04% of total	
Triiodothyroxine (T3)	5481545	230–660 ng/100mL	3.54–10.2 pmol/L
Thyroid-stimulating hormone (TSH)	4854515	2–3.7 µE/mL	2–3.7 mME/L
Protein-bound iodine	1845421	3–7 µg/100mL	0.24–0.55 µmol/L

Table 36

Biogenic Amines – 4148214

Determination	Restorative Sequence	Units	SI-Units
1	2	3	4
Catecholamines in urine: Adrenaline	148542192 1854215	17,5 ± 1,6mkg/s (0,5 - 34,5mkg/s)	32,5 ± 2,2nmol7s (2,7 - 188,4 nmol/s)
Noradrenaline	8214854	36,4 ± 6,6mkg/s (0 - 81,4mkg/s)	76,6 ± 6,3nmol/s (0 - 481,1nmol/s)
Dopamine	5821545	194,0 ± 16,0mkg/s (18,5 - 370,0mkg/s)	487,0 ± 36,9nmol/s (121,4 - 2425nmol/s)

1	2	3	4
Vanillylmandelic acid (VMA)	514821478	0 - 7,5mg/s (2,9 ± 0,3mg/s)	0 - 37,0µmol/s (14,3 ± 1,5µmol/s)
Homovanillic acid	5148215	2,9 ± 0,2mg/s (0,5 - 4,6mg/s)	16,1 ± 0,8µmol/s (7,1 - 25,1µmol/s)
5-Hydroxyindoleacetic acid (HIAA)	1854212	2 - 3,9mg/s	10,7 - 20,5µmol/s
Serotonin, blood	5148123	0,1 - 0,3mkg/ml	340 - 1100µmol/s
Histamine, blood	514854291	0,02 - 0,07mkg7ml	539 - 899µmol/s

Table 37

OTHER HORMONES – 518214831

Determination	Restorative Sequence	Units	SI-Units
Growth hormone (GH):	514821479		
male	54321487	0.025–0.5 mg/mL	0.025–0.5 µg/L
female	5185214	0.081–3.36 mg/mL	0.081–3.36 µg/L
Insulin, blood	5845421	5–20 MED/L	36–143 pmol/L
Gastrin	9990185	20–90 ng/mL	20–90 µg/L
Glucagon, blood, pancreas	5482157	30–120 ng/mL	30–120 ng/L
C-peptide, blood	45481422	1.0–4.5 ng/mL	1–4.5 µg/L

Appendix I

Concentration on Eight-Digit Numbers

Diagnosis	Concentration-Number	Page
Appendicitis, acute – 54321484		140(32)
Enteritis, acute – 54321481		71(22)
Hepatitis, acute – 58432141		66(24)
Upper respiratory tract infection – 48145488		96(20)
Laryngitis, allergic – 58143214		105(01)
Pneumonitis, hypersensitive – 51843215		106(04)
Allergic alveolitis – 51843215		106(04)
Anemia – 48543212		75(14)
Aneurysm – 48543218		140(26)
Heart defects, congenital –14891548		103(23)
Occlusion of major arteries – 81543213		146(32)
Asthma bronchiale – 58145428		101(01)
Atherosclerosis – 54321898		47(22)
Coronary heart disease – 54321898		47(22)
Ectopia lentis (Lens displacement) – 25184321		161(04)
Bartholinitis – 58143215		116(01)
Bauhinitis – 58432148		68(22)
Ileocecal valve inflammation – 58432148		68(22)
Bronchiolitis – 89143215		56(26)
Bronchiole, acute inflammation of – 89143215		56(26)
Pityriasis versicolor – 18543214		137(09)
Bursitis – 75184321		152(30)
Candidiasis – 54842148		61(03)
Thrush – 54842148		61(03)

Cerumen – 48145814	155(05)
Earwax – 48145814	155(05)
Pneumonia, chronic – 51421543	105(27)
Dacryocystitis – 45184321	161(01)
Hypopituitarism – 48143214	82(06)
Panhypopituitarism – 48143214	82(06)
Simmond's disease – 48143214	82(06)
Diverticulum – 48543217	142(33)
Dyskinesia, biliary – 58432144	63(07)
Dyskinesia, intestines – 54321893	63(11)
Adie syndrome – 18543211	120(13)
Mydrisasis – 18543211	120(13)
Pupillotonia – 18543211	120(13)
Cystadenoma, ovarian – 58432143	116(20)
Ulcer (simple) of the small intestine – 48481452	71(13)
Anemia, toxic hemolytic – 45481424	100(33)
Osteomyelitis, epiphyseal – 12345895	110(30)
Hypogalactia – 48123147	112(29)
Lactation disorder – 48123147	112(29)
Occupational diseases, through the influence of biological factors – 81432184	84(19)
Cervical erosion – 54321459	116(07)
Ectropion, cervical – 54321459	116(07)
Erythema nodosum – 15184321	135(19)
Eustachitis – 18554321	155(12)
Enteropathy, exudative – 48123454	64(08)
Favism – 54321457	76(26)
Foreign bodies, ear – 54321545	155(15)
Foreign bodies, esophagus – 14854321	144(07)
Dyskinesia of the digestive tract – 81234574	63(01)
Dyspepsia – 81234574	63(01)
Diarrhea, functional – 81234574	63(01)
Jaundice, functional – 84514851	69(05)
Hyperbilirubinemia, benign – 84514851	67(31)
Galactosemia – 48125421	103(16)

Gas gangrene – 41543218	144(28)
Gastroptosis – 81234574	63(01)
Herpes zoster – 51454322	122(24)
Shingles – 51454322	122(24)
Hemoblastosis outside of bone marrow, Hematosarcoma, and Lymphoma – 54321451	77(01)
Lymphocytoma – 54321451	41(23)
Hemorrhagic diathesis, caused by pathology of the blood vessels – 54815438	77(11)
Hemorrhoids – 58143219	145(11)
Cancer, bladder – 89123459	38(10)
Hepatocerebral dystrophy – 48143212	122(17)
Wilson's disease – 48143212	122(17)
Ptosis – 18543121	163(26)
Upper eyelid, drooping – 18543121	163(26)
Hernia – 95184321	145(14)
Hydrocephalus – 81432143	122(28)
Hymenolepiasis – 54812548	91(21)
Dwarf tapeworm infestation – 54812548	91(21)
Hyperinsulinemia – 48454322	81(23)
Dysinsulinism – 48454322	81(23)
Hypogonadism (male) – 48143121	81(33)
Cushing's syndrome – 54321458	80(21)
Itsenko Cushing – 54321458	80(21)
Catatonia – 51843214	128(29)
Cat scratch disease – 48145421	88(18)
Lymphadenitis, subacute regional – 48145421	88(18)
Cephalohematoma – 48543214	109(34)
Cramps – 51245424	101(18)
Spasms – 51245424	104(24)
Kraurosis vulvae – 58143218	117(13)
Circulatory failure – 85432102	48(23)
Labyrinthitis – 48154219	155(31)
Leiomyoma – 55114214	146(01)
Emphysema – 54321892	57(08)

Pulmonary infarction – 89143211	58(21)
Lung infarction – 89143211	58(21)
Pulmonary edema – 54321112	51(01)
Lung edema – 54321112	51(01)
Pyloric stenosis – 81543211	148(25)
Mastopathy – 84854321	146(18)
Meningitis –51485431	122(33)
Mesothelioma – 58912434	42(08)
Metagonimiasis – 54812541	92(29)
Crohn's disease – 94854321	141(33)
Multiple Sclerosis – 51843218	123(07)
Myelopathia – 51843219	123(24)
Myocarditis – 85432104	50(21)
Narcolepsy – 48543216	124(05)
Epistaxis – 65184321	155(08)
Nose bleeds – 65184321	155(08)
Neurotic disorder – 48154211	130(15)
Cancer, kidney – 56789108	39(12)
Postnatal and postpartum period (lasts 6 plus weeks) – 12891451	114(01)
Esophagitis – 54321489	64(30)
Otitis (externa, media, interna) – 55184321	156(28)
Parkinson's disease – 54811421	124(29)
Peridontal disease – 58145421	167(01)
Pathologische postnatale Periode – 41854218	114(04)
Lice, infestation of – 48148121	93(28)
Polyarteritis nodosa – 54321894	54(13)
Periarteritis nodosa – 54321894	54(13)
Kussmaul disease – 54321894	54(13)
Phlegmon – 48143128	147(29)
Phlegmon, newborns – 51485433	111(01)
Pneumatosis, gastric – 54321455	70(01)
Portal Hypertension – 45143211	106(11)
Psychosis, presenile – 18543219	131(14)
Muscular dystrophy, progressive – 85432183	123(12)

Psychoorganic syndrome – 51843212   131(01)
Pterygium – 18543212   163(23)
Surfer's eye – 18543212   163(23)
Pyelonephritis – 58143213   73(10)
Pyoderma – 51432149   137(25)
Allergies, respiratory – 45143212   100(18)
Anal canal, tears or cracks in – 81454321   140(22)
Tumor, spinal cord – 51843210   44(01)
Sarcoma, soft tissue – 54321891   42(31)
Brain injury, traumatic – 51843213   121(04)
Liver damage – 48145428   86(19)
Hepatopathy, toxic – 48145428   86(19)
Schistosomiasis – 48125428   94(33)
Bilharziosis – 48125428   94(33)
Strongyloidiasis – 54812527   95(04)
Malabsorption – 48543215   69(20)
Tonsillitis, chronic – 35184321   158(27)
Encephalopathy, traumatic – 18543217   129(01)
Colitis, ulcerative – 48143211   141(25)
Myoma, uterine – 51843216   117(31)
Varicocele – 81432151   150(08)
Ovalocytosis, hereditary – 51454323   78(09)
Elliptocytosis, hereditary – 51454323   78(09)
Encephalitis, viral – 48188884   121(29)
Virilism – 89143212   83(04)
Varicella (Chickenpox) – 48154215   96(25)
Hypoplasia, tooth enamel – 74854321   166(16)
Zinga – 54321481   71(22)
Cystitis – 48543211   72(16)

Table in Chpt. 26   169
    Restorative Number Sequences for Unknown
    Diagnoses, Diseases and Conditions – Neck – 18548321

NORMAL LABORATORY TEST VALUES   170

Table 1. Peripheral Blood   171
   Hemoglobin: male – 81432142
   Erythrocytes: male – 81543212
   Pigment content – 81432152

Table 2. Erythrocytes   172
   Osmotic resistance of erythrocytes
   Minimum – 18543210
   Maximum – 58432142

Table 2. Thrombocytogram   173
   Thrombocytes: young – 18543213

Table 6. Coagulation and Fibrinolytic Activity
   of the Blood   175
   Coagulation time – 51432141
   Bleeding time – 51454328
   Plasma recalcification time – 51485432

Table 6. Coagulation and Fibrinolytic Activity
   of the Blood   176
   Plasma fibrinogen B test – 14814325
   Factor X Concentration – 45481451
   Factor VIII (proconvertin) – 54321483

Table 8. Physical Characteristics – 85432181   177

Table 9. Chemical Constituents of Urine   177
   pH Reaction – 51432181
   Protein – 54321858

Table 10. Stool Microscopy   180
   Leukocytes – 82143213

Table 10. Stool Microscopy   180
   Amount – 18754321
   pH – 14542108

Table 11. Chemical Constituents of Saliva – 14542101   181
   Protein – 54854321
   Urea – 54815425

Table 12. Gastric Juice (Empty Stomach) – 48142123   182
   Gastric juice specimens are collected In a fasted
   state in intervals
   of 15 min – 81454322
   Free Hydrochloric acid, hourly – 54321482

Table 12. Stimulants of Gastric Secretion – 12345717   183

Table 15. Bile Acid Stimulation   185
   Relative density – 89143214

Table 17. Cerebrospinal Fluid   185
   Pressure, lying – 52143213

Table 18. Protein and Protein   186
   Fractions – 185843218
   Fibrinogen – 58432149

Table 20. Rest Nitrogen and its
   Components – 91854321   187

Table 20. Xanthoproteic reaction – 54321488   188

Table 22. Content of the Blood Plasma   189
   Triglycerides (blood serum) – 18543215

Table 24. Lipoproteids in the Blood Serum   190
Cholesterol (total) – 51245422

Table 26. Bilirubin Metabolism in Blood   191
Unconjugated bilirubin (BU) – 52143218

Table 27. Electrolytes and Trace Minerals in the Blood   192
Transferrin, free – 18543216

Table 33. Hypophyseal-Gonadotropic Hormones   196
Progesterone ng/mL – 51421541

Table 35. Thyroid Hormones – 81432157   197

Table 37. Other Hormones   198
Growth hormone (GH): male – 54321487
C-peptide, blood – 45481422

Appendix II

Concentration on Nine-Digit Numbers

Diagnosis Concentration	Number	Page
Adrenogenital syndrome – 148542121		115(26)
Aerosinusitis – 514854237		154(17)
Sinus barotrauma – 514854237		154(17)
Affective disorder – 548142182		128(10)
Duodenitis, acute – 481543288		62(23)
Mastoiditis, acute – 514832186		156(11)
Tracheitis, allergic – 514854218		108(19)
Amenorrhea – 514354832		115(30)
Congenital cholangiopathy of the newborn – 948514211		150(25)
Atresia, biliary – 948514211		150(25)
Hernia, congenital diaphragmatic – 518543257		151(17)
Ankylosis, TMJ (temporomandibular joint) – 514852179		167(28)
Aspergillosis – 481543271		56(17)
Sebaceous cyst – 888888179		149(01)
Steatoma – 888888179		149(01)
Brill-Zinsser disease – 514854299		88(07)
Cheilitis – 518431482		165(21)
Chapped lips – 518431482		165(21)
Deformations, nasal septal – 148543285		155(01)
Diencephalic syndrome – 514854215		121(25)
Hypothalamic syndrome – 514854215		121(25)
Myotonic dystrophy – 481543244		123(33)
Curschmann-Batten-Steiner syndrome – 481543244		123(33)

Eczema – 548132151	135(10)
Endophthalmitis – 514254842	161(14)
Epiduritis – 888888149	121(32)
Musculoskeletal system, diseases in newborns – 514218873	151(32)
Erythema multiforme – 548142137	135(15)
Foreign bodies, soft tissue – 148543297	144(11)
Vernal keratoconjunctivitis – 514258951	164(21)
Catarrh, spring – 514258951	164(21)
Sclerosis, spinal – 518543251	122(05)
Funicular myelitis – 518543251	122(05)
Putnam-Dana syndrome – 518543251	122(05)
Prolapse, uterus and vagina – 514832183	118(25)
Hordeolum – 514854249	161(31)
Stye – 514854249	161(31)
Acne vulgaris – 514832185	134(11)
Gingivitis – 548432123	166(04)
Glossalgia – 514852181	166(07)
Tongue pain – 514852181	166(07)
Hemophilia – 548214514	104(01)
Tuberculosis, cutaneous – 148543296	139(01)
Hydrocele, testis or spermatic cord – 481543255	145(22)
Intracranial birth injury – 518999981	104(29)
Carbuncle – 483854381	141(09)
Granuloma, esophagus – 148543283	156(01)
Keratitis – 518432114	162(07)
Cyst, jaw – 514218877	165(24)
Talipes equinovarus – 485143241	149(04)
Clubfoot – 485143241	149(04)
Tuberculosis, bone – 148543281	149(23)
Vertigo – 514854217	127(09)
Dizziness – 514854217	127(09)
Cryptorchidism – 485143287	142(05)
Myopia – 548132198	162(09)
Nearsightedness – 548132198	162(09)

Laryngospasm – 485148248	156(07)
Leprosy – 148543294	136(04)
Leukoplakia – 485148151	166(22)
Lymphangitis – 484851482	146(12)
Bipolar disorder – 514218857	128(24)
Manic-depressive disorder – 514218857	128(24)
Rectal prolapse – 514832187	148(33)
Mastocytosis – 148542171	136(23)
Pregnancy, multiple (pregnancy with two or more fetuses) – 123457854	114(21)
Meniere's disease – 514854233	156(15)
Molluscum contagiosum – 514321532	136(26)
Phlegmon, necrotic in newborns – 514852173	152(14)
Neuropathy, facial nerves – 518999955	124(10)
Neuroma, acoustic – 518999955	124(10)
Orchiepididymitis – 818432151	147(01)
Otomycosis – 514832188	157(01)
Ozaena – 514854241	157(08)
Rhinitis, atrophic – 514854241	157(08)
Empyema, pleural – 514854223	143(10)
Pleuritis, purulent – 514854223	143(10)
Polyps, cervical or uterine – 518999973	118(16)
Post-lumbar puncture syndrome – 818543231	125(21)
Paralysis, progressive – 512143223	130(27)
Yersinia pseudotuberculosis – 514854212	97(04)
Psoriasis – 999899181	137(21)
Pyopneumothorax – 148543299	148(30)
Genitals, tears in external genitals – 148543291	114(34)
Rosacea – 518914891	138(04)
Sleep disorder – 514248538	125(30)
Psychosis, senile – 481854383	131(24)
Scleritis, Episcleritis – 514854248	164(01)
Zollinger-Ellison syndrome – 148543295	150(19)
Pneumothorax, spontaneous – 481854221	147(32)
Papilledema (Optic nerve edema) – 145432152	163(11)

Erectile dysfunction – 184854281	132(14)
Strabismus (Tropia, Cross-eyed squint) – 518543254	164(06)
Radiation sickness, acute – 481543294	78(26)
Polycystic Ovarian Disease (Stein-Leventhal syndrome) – 518543248	118(11)
Grandiosity – 148454283	129(06)
Arthritis, TMJ (temporomandibular joint) – 548432174	167(33)
Skin reaction, toxic – 514832184	138(17)
Dyspepsia, toxic – – 514218821	102(27)
Fistula, tracheoesophageal – 514854714	151(12)
Osteomyelitis, traumatic – 514854221	147(04)
Ulcer, tropic – 514852154	149(34)
Tumor, peripheral nervous system – 514832182	43(31)
Ulcer, corneal – 548432194	164(13)
Uveitis – 548432198	164(18)
Rhinitis, vasomotor or allergic – 514852351	157(26)
Pollinosis – 514852351	157(26)
Hay fever – 514852351	157(26)
Dystonia, vegetative-circulatory – 514218838	102(31)
Eyeball injuries – 518432118	161(22)
Occlusion, central retinal artery – 514852178	162(21)
Tooth, fractured (broken) – 814454251	168(09)
Tooth luxation – 485143277	168(05)
Dental calculus – 514852182	165(27)
Dental tartar – 514852182	165(27)
Cyst, bronchial cleft – 514854214	142(08)
Cyst, lateral neck – 514854214	142(08)
Pharyngeal fistula – 514854214	142(08)

Table in Chpt. 26. Restorative Number Sequences
for Unknown Diagnoses, Diseases and Conditions   169
Left Leg – 485148291

NORMAL LABORATORY TEST VALUES   170

Table 1. Peripheral Blood 171
    Erythrocytes – 518432129
    Leukocytes – 514854240
    Leukocytes: male – 514852187

Table 1. Peripheral Blood 171
    Reticulocytes – 518231418
    ESR (Erythrocyte Sedimentation Rate) – 514832101
    ESR (Erythrocyte Sedimentation Rate): male – 514254351
    Hematocrit – HCT (percentage of blood comprised of
    red blood cells) – 148542118

Table 2. Differential Leukocyte Count 172
    Neutrophils (granulocytes) – 485148293
    Neutrophils (granulocytes): banded – 514832102
    Neutrophils (granulocytes): segmented – 518432128
    Basophils (granulocytes) – 518432120
    Monocytes – 514232191

Table 2. Erythrocytes 172
    Osmotic resistance of erythrocytes – 148542145
    Incubated blood, average – 518543299

Table 2. Thrombocytogram 172
    Old – 514858451
    Degenerative form – 514853258
    With vacuolization – 514231481

Table 3. Cytology, Bone Marrow Aspirate (Sternum) 173
    Cell Types – 514321541
    Neutrophil: Promyelocytes – 514254355
    Myelocytes – 518432125
    Metamyelocytes: banded – 514231482
    Metamyelocytes: segmented – 514832103

Table 3. Cytology, Bone Marrow Aspirate (Sternum) 174
    Pronormoblasts (Pronormocytes) – 518432123
    Normoblasts (Normocytes) – 518432124
    basophil – 548432125
    polychromatophilic – 514832108
    orthochromatic – 518432122
    Plasma cells – 518432134
    Reticular cells – 518432137
    Megakaryocytes – 514832107
    Leuko-erythroblastic ratio – 148542199
    Maturation: Erythrokaryocytes – 548451238
    Maturation: Neutrophil – 514832105

Table 4. Morphological Cytology, Lymph Node,
    Calculation per 1000 Cells 174
    Prolymphocytes – 518432135
    Monocytes – 548432188
    Mast cells – 543218823

Table 5. Morphological Cytology, Spleen,
    Calculation per 1000 Cells 175
    Myelocytes – 514832191
    Metamyelocytes – 584321591
    Neutrophil granulocytes – 548132174

Table 6. Coagulation and Fibrinolytic Activity
    of the Blood – 751483218 175
    Thromboelastography (TEG)– 514832193
    Reaction time (R) – 548543234

Table 6. Coagulation and Fibrinolytic Activity
    of the Blood – 751483218 176
    Prothrombin time capillary blood – 514231499
    Antithrombin activity – 514852191

Plasma fibrinogen – Factor 1
(calorimetric method) – 514832192
Factor XIII (fibrin stabilizing factor) – 485142175
Thromboplastin generation test
(Plasma, Thrombocytes, Serum) – 514832194
Factor V (accelerator globulin) – 548132132
Plasma soluble fibrin monomer complex – 518432132

Table 7. ABO System Forward Typing with Serum
(containing antibodies) – 148542117   176
O (I) – 148542188
A (II) – 145432171

Table 8. ABO System Back Typing (patient's
blood serum is mixed with standard Erythrocytes)   177
Oaß (I) – 148542185
Aß (II) – 145432182

Table 9. Chemical Constituents of Urine   177
Acetone – 543218848
Uric acid – 518888842
Creatinine: male – 814254351
Creatine – 518432139
Uropepsin – 518432179

Table 9. Urine Sediment   178
Leukocytes: female – 543218845
Bacteria – 514831254
Inorganic sediment – 514218878

Table 9. Urine Analysis Methods   179
Kakowski-Addis Method – 514218897
In 24 hr urine collection: casts – 514548823
Nechiporenko Method – 148851481
In 1 mL urine:: Erythrocytes – 514548891

Table 10. Instestinal Contents 180
    Consistency – 148543287
    Form – 148543290
    Color – 512314542
    Mucus, blood – 518432181

Table 10. Stool Microscopy 180
    Cell tissue – 518432183
    Fats – 518432187
    Fatty acids, fatty soaps – 145432191
    Vegetable fiber – 518432189

Table 10. Chemical Constituents of the
Intestinal Contents 180
    Fats – 548214583
    Urobilin – 148542183

Table 11. Saliva – 514821441 181

Table 11. Chemical Constituents of Saliva 181
    Chloride – 514852193

Table 12. Chemical Constituents of the Gastric Juice 182
    Non-protein nitrogen – 814854218
    Urea and ammonia – 548214891
    Uric acid – 514832198

Table 12. Gastric Juice (Empty Stomach) 182
    Amount – 514854148
    Free Hydrochloric acid – 518432191
    Hydrochloric acid, hourly – 514254481

Table 13. Stimulated Gastric Secretion – 148542173 183
    Free Hydrogen chloride – 148542177

Table 13. Microscopy of the Stomach Contents 183
    Epithel – 548543281
    Erythrocytes – 514854251
    Leukocytes – 518432199
    Yeast – 514854258
    Lactobacillus – 518432197

Table 14. Bile – 514852188 184

Table 14. Composition of Bile (g/L) 184
    Choline – 518432198
    Protein – 514821447
    Trypsin – 514854261

Table 14. Evaluation of Duodenal
    Contents – 215184321 184

Table 16. Microscopic Examination of the
    Bile Specimens 185
    Leukocytes in the visual field – 235184321
    Mucus – 148542175

Table 17. Cerebrospinal Fluid 185
    pH – 514821453
    Protein (total) – 775184321

Table 18. Biochemistry of the Blood – 514832189 186

Table 18. Protein and Protein Fractions 186
    Albumin – 815184321

Table 19. Protein Fractions
    (Paper Electrophoresis) – 148542138 187

Table 20. Rest Nitrogen and its Components   187
     Amino acid nitrogen – 148542161
     Uric acid – 815518432
     Creatine – 885184321
     Creatine: male – 295184321
     Ammonia – 489152141

Table 21. Amino Acids Blood Plasma   188
     Valine – 518254442

Table 22. Content of the Blood Plasma   188
     Non-esterified fatty acid – 145454577
     High-density Lipoprotein (HDL)
     α-Lipoprotein (25 – 30%): female – 542143221
     Low-density Lipoprotein (LDL)
     ß-Lipoprotein (65 – 75%) – 174845421

Table 23. Total Cholesterol in Relation to Age   188
     40 – 543218891

Table 24. Lipoproteids in the Blood Serum   189
     Phosphor lipids (%) – 514854272

Table 25. Carbohydrate Metabolism of
     the Blood – 514214891   190
     Glycogen – 785184321

Table 25. Carbohydrate Metabolism of
     the Blood – 514214891   191
     O-Toluidine method – 148542163
     Plasma – 548214547

Table 26. Bilirubin Metabolism in Blood – 548132177   191

Table 27. Electrolytes and Trace Minerals in

the Blood – 518431181   192
Magnesium, serum – 514831298
Lithium – 514821458

Table 28. Blood pH   192
Buffer base – (BB) – 514821461
Bicarbonate – 555184321

Table 28. Blood Enzymes   193
Amylase – 148542114
Aspartate transaminase (SGOT) – 148582114
Trypsin – 148542187

Table 28. Immunological Blood Values – 148542153   194
Cancer antigens – 481854224

Table 31. Hormone Content in the Blood   195
Adrenocorticotropic hormone (ACTH) – 148542191

Table 33. Hypophyseal-Gonadotropic Hormones   196
Hormone: Luteinizing hormone (LH),
hormone/mL – 514852199
DHEA, mg/s – 514821465

Table 36. Biogenic Amines   197
Catecholamines in urine – 148542192

Table 36. Biogenic Amines   198
Vanillylmandelic acid (VMA) – 514821478
Histamine, blood – 514854291

Table 37. Other Hormones – 518214831   198
Growth hormone (GH) – 514821479

Index

A

Abdomen, acute – 5484543	140(12)
Abdominal cavity,	
surgical diseases of organs of – 5184311	150(29)
Abdominal typhus – 1411111	96(04)
Abruption, placental – 1111155	113(25)
Abscess – 8148321	140(15)
Abscess, cerebral – 1894811	120(10)
Abscess, premaxillary – 518231415	165(10)
Abscess, retropharyngeal – 1454321	154(10)
Achalasia of cardia – 4895132	60(10)
Achylia gastrica – 8432157	60(20)
Acne vulgaris – 514832185	134(11)
Acoustic, neuroma – 518999955	124(10)
Acromegaly – 1854321	80(10)
Actinomycosis – 4832514	140(18)
Actinomycosis of the skin – 148542156	134(15)
Addison's disease – 4812314	80(15)
Adenoids – 5189514	154(13)
Adie syndrome – 18543211	120(13)
Adnexitis, fallopian tube – 5148914	118(33)
Adnexitis, ovary – 5143548	117(34)
Adrenal hyperplasia, congenital – 45143213	100(10)
Adrenal insufficiency – 4812314	80(16)
Adrenogenital syndrome – 148542121	115(26)
Aerosinusitis – 514854237	154(17)

Affective disorder – 548142182 — 128(10)
Agranulocytosis – 4856742 — 75(10)
AIDS – 5148555 — 91(13)
Alcoholism – 148543292 — 128(17)
Alimentary dystrophy – 5456784 — 70(29)
Allergic diathesis – 0195451 — 100(14)
Allergic vasculitis – 8491234 — 53(28)
Allergies, respiratory – 45143212 — 100(18)
Alopecia – 5484121 — 134(18)
Alpha 1-antitrypsin deficiency – 1454545 — 100(22)
Alport syndrome – 5854312 — 105(18)
Alveolitis, allergic – 51843215 — 106(04)
Alveolitis, dental – 5848188 — 165(14)
Alveolococcosis – 5481454 — 87(10)
Amblyopia – 1899999 — 160(10)
Amenorrhea – 514354832 — 115(30)
Amnesia – 4185432 — 129(23)
Amniocele – 5143248 — 110(25)
Amniotic fluid embolism – 5123412 — 112(11)
Amoebiasis – 1289145 — 87(14)
Amputation, traumatic – 5451891 — 152(23)
Amyloidosis – 4512345 — 72(11)
Amyloidosis – 5432185 — 160(27)
Amyotrophic lateral sclerosis – 5148910 — 120(17)
Anal fissure – 81454321 — 140(22)
Anemia – 48543212 — 75(14)
Anemia – 48543212 — 100(26)
    aplastic – 5481541 — 75(21)
    autoimmune hemolytic – 5814311 — 75(27)
    congenital – 4581254 — 75(31)
    hemolytic – 5484813 — 76(03)
    hypoplastic – 5481541 — 75(21)
    iron deficiency – 1458421 — 100(28)
    lead poisoning, from – 1237819 — 75(17)
    megaloblastic – 5481254 — 76(06)

posthemorrhagic acute – 9481232	76(11)
sickle-cell – 7891017	76(15)
sideroblastic – 4581254	75(31)
toxic hemolytic – 45481424	100(33)
Aneurysm – 48543218	140(26)
Aneurysm, cerebral – 1485999	120(23)
Angiitis, cutaneous – 1454231	139(20)
Angina pectoris – 8145999	51(10)
Angina tonsillaris – 1999999	154(21)
Angiofibroma, nasopharyngeal juvenile – 1111122	154(25)
Angioma – 4812599	109(12)
Ankylosis – 1848522	152(27)
Ankylostomiasis – 4815454	87(20)
Anovulatory cycle – 4813542	115(33)
Anthracosis – 5843214	56(10)
Anthrax – 9998991	87(24)
Antisocial personality disorder – 4182546	131(04)
Apoplexy	
ovarian – 1238543	118(03)
spinal – 8888881	126(04)
stroke – 4818542	126(07)
Appendicitis, acute – 54321484	140(32)
Appendicitis, childhood – 9999911	109(15)
Arachnoiditis – 4567549	120(28)
Arrhythmia – 8543210	47(17)
Arteritis – giant-cell cranial, or temporal – 9998102	53(16)
Arthritis	
degenerative – 8145812	52(17)
infectious – 8111110	53(33)
reactive – 4848111	52(23)
rheumatoid – 8914201	52(28)
Arthritis psoriatica – 0145421	52(13)
Arthrosis deformans – 8145812	52(17)
Asbestosis – 4814321	56(14)
Ascariasis – 4814812	87(27)

Ascorbic acid deficiency – 4141255 — 99(21)
Aspergillosis – 481543271 — 56(17)
Asphyxia, fetal – 4812348 — 112(16)
Asphyxia, newborn – 4812348 — 112(16)
Asthenia – 1891013 — 120(32)
Asthenopia – 9814214 — 160(14)
Asthma bronchiale, childhood – 58145428 — 101(01)
Asthma cardiale – 8543214 — 48(01)
Asthma, bronchial – 8943548 — 56(22)
Astigmatism – 1421543 — 160(17)
Atherosclerosis – 54321898 — 47(22)
Athetosis – 1454891 — 121(01)
Atresia
    anal and rectal – 6555557 — 109(22)
    biliary – 948514211 — 150(25)
    biliary in childhood – 9191918 — 109(25)
    choanal – 1989142 — 154(28)
    duodenal – 5557777 — 109(19)
    esophageal – 8194321 — 109(28)
    esophagus – 518543157 — 151(03)
    small intestine – 9188888 — 109(31)
Auricular hematoma – 4853121 — 156(23)
Autonomic neuropathy – 8432910 — 47(29)
Avitaminosis – 5451234 — 98(10)

B

Bacteriosis, E. coli – 1238888 — 89(15)
Balanoposthitis – 5814231 — 134(22)
Balantidiasis – 1543218 — 87(31)
Baldness – 5484121 — 134(18)
Bang's disease – 4122222 — 88(10)
Bartholinitis – 58143215 — 116(01)
Basedow's disease – 5143218 — 81(15)
Bauhinitis – 58432148 — 68(22)

Bechterew's disease – 4891201	55(06)
Bed sores – 6743514	142(21)
Bee stings – 9189189	86(06)
Bell's palsy – 518999955	124(10)
Beriberi – 3489112	60(34)
Bilharziosis – 48125428	94(33)
Bipolar disorder – 514218857	128(24)
Birth, preterm – 1284321	114(31)
Black lung disease – 8148545	57(03)
Bladder infection – 48543211	72(16)
Bleeding	
during childbirth – 4814821	112(20)
dysfunctional bleeding of the uterus – 4853541	117(04)
external – 4321511	145(01)
gastrointestinal – 5121432	110(07)
internal – 5142543	145(06)
nasal septum – 5431482	155(28)
tooth extraction, after – 8144542	165(18)
Bleeding diathesis – 5148543	77(08)
Blepharitis – 5142589	160(20)
Blistering disease – 8145321	137(01)
Blood cancer – 5481347	77(20)
Blood loss, acute – 9481232	76(11)
Blood poisoning, acute – 8914321	45(10)
Blood poisoning, chronic – 8145421	45(10)
Boil – 5148385	144(25)
Botkin's disease – 5412514	91(01)
Botulism, foodborne – 5481252	88(04)
Brain abscess – 1894811	120(10)
Brain injury, traumatic – 51843213	121(04)
Brill-Zinsser disease – 514854299	88(07)
Bronchiectasis – 4812578	141(01)
Bronchioles, acute inflammation of – 89143215	56(26)
Bronchiolitis – 89143215	56(26)

Bronchitis
        acute – 4812567   56(31)
        acute (childhood) – 5482145   101(06)
        allergic – 5481432   101(09)
        chronic – 4218910   56(34)
Bronze diabetes – 5454589   61(01)
Brucellosis – 4122222   88(10)
Bruise – 0156912   141(30)
Buerger's disease – 5432142   149(08)
Buerger's disease – 8945482   55(24)
Bulging eye – 5454311   161(18)
Bunion – 5418521   153(04)
Burns, thermal – 8191111   141(05)
Bursitis – 75184321   152(30)
Bursitis (see Rheumatism, soft tissue) – 1489123   54(33)

C

Campylobacter jejuni – 4815421   88(14)
Cancer
        bile duct – 5891248   39(19)
        bladder – 89123459   38(10)
        bone – 1234589   38(14)
        breast – 5432189   38(20)
        colon – 5821435   38(26)
        esophageal – 8912567   38(33)
        external genitals – 2589121   41(16)
        extrahepatic bile duct – 5789154   39(01)
        gallbladder – 8912453   39(06)
        gastric – 8912534   40(32)
        hepatic – 5891248   39(19)
        kidney – 56789108   39(12)
        lips – 1567812   39(16)
        liver – 5891248   39(19)
        lung – 4541589   58(12)

major duodenal papilla – 8912345	39(27)
mouth and throat – 1235689	39(32)
ovarian – 4851923	40(01)
pancreatic – 8125891	40(05)
penis – 8514921	40(10)
prostate – 4321890	40(13)
salivary gland – 9854321	40(17)
skin – 8148957	40(21)
small intestines – 5485143	40(28)
stomach – 8912534	40(32)
testicular – 5814321	41(03)
thyroid – 5814542	41(08)
ureter – 5891856	41(12)
vaginal – 2589121	41(16)
vulva – 5148945	41(20), 116(04)
Candidiasis – 54842148	61(03)
Candidiasis – 9876591	134(25)
Candidiasis of the lung – 4891444	58(16)
Canicola fever – 5128432	92(04)
Carboconiosis – 8148545	57(03)
Carbuncle – 483854381	141(09)
Carcinoid syndrome – 4848145	61(07)
Carcinoma, cholangio – 5891248	39(19)
Carcinoma, hepatocellular – 5891248	39(19)
Cardiac aneurysm – 9187549	141(12)
Cardiac arrest – 8915678	36(10)
Cardiac asthma – 8543214	48(01)
Cardiac dysrhythmia – 8543210	47(17)
Cardiac failure – 8542196	49(23)
Cardiac sphincter, insufficiency of – 8545142	68(29)
Cardialgia – 8124567	48(06)
Cardiogenic (shock – 1895678	36(17)
Cardiomyopathy – 8421432	48(11)
Cardiosclerosis – 4891067	48(18)

Cardiospasm – 4895132   60(07)
Cardiovascular insufficiency, acute – 1895678   36(17)
Caries, teeth – 5148584   165(30)
Cat scratch disease – 48145421   88(18)
Cataract – 5189142   160(23)
Catatonia – 51843214   128(29)
Cauliflower ear – 4853121   156(23)
Celiac disease – 4154548   101(15)
Celiac sprue – 4891483   64(12)
Cephalgia – 4818543   122(10)
Cephalohematoma – 48543214   109(34)
Cerebral palsy – 4818521   121(08)
Cerebroside lipoidosis – 5145432   76(31)
Cerebrovascular insult – 4818542   126(07)
Cerumen – 48145814   155(05)
Cervical erosion – 54321459   116(07)
Chalazion – 5148582   160(26)
Chancroid – 4815451   139(08)
Chapped lips – 518431482   165(21)
Charcot-Marie-Tooth disease – 4814512   121(13)
Cheilitis – 518431482   165(21)
Chemotherapy, side effects of – 4812813   76(20)
Chickenpox – 48154215   96(25)
Choking – 4821543   103(12)
Cholangiopathy of the newborn, congenital
    – 948514211   150(25)
Cholangitis – 8431548   141(15)
Cholecystitis, acute – 4154382   141(18)
Cholecystitis, chronic – 5481245   61(16)
Cholecystolithiasis – 0148012   141(21)
Cholera – 4891491   88(22)
Cholestasis – 5421548   67(15)
Chorea – 4831485   121(18)
Choriocarcinoma – 4854123   116(11)
Chorioiditis – 5182584   160(29)

Chorionepithelioma – 4854123	116(11)
Chronic fatigue syndrome – 1891013	120(32)
Circulatory failure – 85432102	48(23)
Cirrhosis of the liver – 4812345	61(22)
Cleft palate – 5151515	110(33)
Climacteric, female – 4851548	117(27)
Clonorchiasis – 5412348	88(25)
Clubfoot – 485143241	149(04)
Cluster headache – 4851485	122(13)
Coagulopathy, consumptive – 8123454	46(11)
Coal worker's pneumoconiosis – 8148545	57(03)
Cold sores – 2312489	91(08)
Colitis	
acute – 5432145	61(32)
chronic – 5481238	62(01)
colitis – 8454321	61(30)
ulcerative – 48143211	141(25)
Collapse – 8914320	48(29)
Colorectal cancer – 5821435	38(26)
Colpitis – 5148533	116(15)
Coma – 1111012	121(22)
Common cold – 48145488	96(20)
Common cold – 5189912	154(32)
Concussion – 51843213	121(04)
Condyloma acuminatum – 1489543	134(30)
Congenital heart defect – 9995437	48(34)
Conjunctivitis – 5184314	160(33)
Conjunctivitis, vernal kerato-c. – 514258951	164(21)
Connective tissue disease, mixed – 1484019	52(33)
Connective tissue diseases, diffuse – 5485812	53(03)
Constipation – 5484548	62(05)
Consumptive coagulopathy – 8123454	46(11)
Contact poisoning – 4814823	85(10)
Contracture, Dupuytren's – 5185421	152(33)
Contracture, joint – 8144855	153(01)

Contusion – 0156912 141(30)
Cor pulmonale – 5432111 49(05)
Coronary heart disease – 1454210 50(05)
Corpus luteum rupture – 1238543 118(03)
Coryza – 5189912 154(32)
Cramps – 51245424 101(18)
Cranial arteritis – 9998102 53(16)
Crohn's disease – 94854321 141(33)
Cross-eyed squint – 518543254 164(06)
Cryptorchidism – 485143287 142(05)
Crystal Deposition Disease Syndrome – 0014235 53(08)
Curschmann-Batten-Steiner syndrome – 481543244 123(33)
Cushing's syndrome – 54321458 80(21)
Cyclothymia – 514218857 128(24)
Cyst
  branchial cleft – 514854214 142(08)
  breast – 4851432 142(13)
  jaw – 514218877 165(24)
  lateral neck – 514854214 142(08)
  median neck – 4548541 142(17)
  mucous – 5148322 156(19)
  ovarian – 5148538 116(17)
  pilonidal – 9018532 143(22)
  thyroglossal – 4548541 142(17)
Cystadenoma, ovarian – 58432143 116(20)
Cystic fibrosis – 9154321 101(22)
Cystic lung disease, congenital – 4851484 151(08)
Cysticercosis – 4512824 88(29)
Cystitis – 48543211 72(16)

D

Dacryocystitis – 45184321 161(01)
De Toni-Debré-Fankoni syndrome – 4514848 101(28)
Decubitus – 6743514 142(21)

Deformations, nasal septal – 148543285	155(01)
Degenerative arthritis – 8145812	52(17)
Delusional disorder – 8142351	128(33)
Demyelination – 51843218	123(07)
Dental calculus – 514852182	165(27)
Dental caries – 5148584	165(30)
Dental focal infection – 514854814	165(34)
Dental tartar – 514852182	165(27)
Dermatitis – 1853121	135(01)
Dermatitis, atopic – 5484215	135(05)
Dermatomyositis – 5481234	53(12)
Diabetes insipidus – 4818888	80(25)
Diabetes insipidus, childhood – 5121111	101(34)
Diabetes mellitus – 4851421	102(04)
Diabetes mellitus – 8819977	80(30)
Diabetes, phosphate – 5148432	102(10)
Diarrhea	
diarrhea – 5843218	62(08)
functional – 81234574	63(01)
tropical – 5481215	70(23)
DIC syndrome – 8123454	46(11)
Diencephalic syndrome – 514854215	121(25)
Dimple, post-anal – 9018532	143(22)
Diphtheria – 5556679	89(01)
Diphyllobothriasis – 4812354	89(07)
Disseminated Intravascular Coagulation – 8123454	46(11)
Distortion – 5148517	153(18)
Diverticulosis, colon – 4851614	142(27)
Diverticulum – 48543217	142(33)
Dizziness – 514854217	127(09)
Drug addiction – 5333353	129(32)
Dry mouth – 5814514	168(17)
Dry socket – 5848188	165(14)
Dumping syndrome (gastric) – 4184214	143(01)
Duodenitis – 5432114	62(20)

Duodenitis, acute – 481543288   62(23)
Duodenitis, chronic – 8432154   62(28)
Duodenum, inflammation of – 5432114   62(20)
Dysbacteriosis, intestinal – 5432101   62(33)
Dysentery – 4812148   89(11)
Dysinsulinism – 48454322   81(23)
Dyskinesia of the digestive tract – 81234574   63(01)
Dyskinesia, biliary – 58432144   63(07)
Dyskinesia, intestines – 54321893   63(11)
Dysmenorrhea – 4815812   116(23)
Dyspepsia
       dyspepsia – 1112223   63(19)
       dyspepsia – 81234574   63(01)
       functional – 5484214   63(24)
       parenteral – 8124321   102(15)
       simple – 5142188   102(20)
       toxic – 514218821   102(27)
Dyspituitarism – 4145412   81(01)
Dystonia, vegetative-circulatory – 514218838   102(31)

E

E. coli bacteriosis – 1238888   89(15)
Ear infection – 55184321   156(28)
Ear wax – 48145814   155(05)
Ebola – 5184599   92(18)
Echinococcosis – 5481235   89(20)
Echinococcosis, alveolar – 5481454   87(10)
Ectopia lentis – 25184321   161(04)
Ectropion – 5142321   161(08)
Ectropion, cervical – 54321459   116(07)
Eczema – 548132151   135(10)
Edema, hunger – 5456784   70(29)
Edema, lung – 54321112   51(01)
Ejaculation disorders – 1482541   132(10)

Electric shock injuries – 5185431 — 143(06)
Elliptocytosis, hereditary – 51454323 — 78(09)
Embolism, amniotic fluid – 5123412 — 112(11)
Emphysema, lung – 54321892 — 57(08)
Empyema, pleural – 514854223 — 143(10)
Encephalitis, tick-borne – 7891010 — 89(24)
Encephalitis, viral – 48188884 — 121(29)
Encephalopathy, traumatic – 18543217 — 129(01)
Endangiitis obliterans – 4518521 — 143(14)
Endocarditis – 8145999 — 49(11)
Endocervicitis – 4857148 — 116(26)
Endometriosis – 5481489 — 116(30)
Endometritis – 8142522 — 116(33)
Endophthalmitis – 514254842 — 161(14)
Enteritis – 8431287 — 63(29)
Enteritis, chronic – 5432140 — 63(32)
Enterobiasis – 5123542 — 89(29)
Enteropathy
    disaccharidase deficiency – 4845432 — 64(03)
    exudative – 48123454 — 64(08)
    gluten-induced – 4891483 — 64(12)
    of the intestines – 8432150 — 64(19)
    protein-losing – 4548123 — 103(01)
Enteroviruses – 8123456 — 89(33)
Enthesopathy (see Rheumatism, soft tissue) – 1489123 — 54(33)
Epidermal necrolyses, toxic – 4891521 — 136(15)
Epidermophyton – 5148532 — 137(28)
Epidural abscess – 888888149 — 121(32)
Epiduritis – 888888149 — 121(32)
Epilepsy – 1484855 — 122(01)
Episcleritis – 514854248 — 164(01)
Epistaxis – 65184321 — 155(08)
Erectile dysfunction – 184854281 — 132(14)
Erysipelas – 4123548 — 90(04)
Erythema multiforme – 548142137 — 135(15)

Erythema nodosum – 15184321   135(19)
Erythrasma – 4821521   135(23)
Erythroblastosis fetalis – 5125432   103(30)
Escherichiosis – 1238888   89(15)
Esophageal spasm – 5481248   64(24)
Esophagitis – 54321489   64(30)
Esophagus
      chemical burn of – 5148599   110(04)
      idiopathic dilation of – 4895132   60(07)
      peptic ulcer – 8432182   65(01)
Eustachitis – 18554321   155(12)
Exophthalmos – 5454311   161(18)
Exotoxic shock – 4185421   86(10)
Exudative enteropathy – 4548123   86(10)
Eye burn – 8881112   162(30)
Eye strain – 9814214   160(14)
Eyeball injuries – 518432118   161(22)
Eyelid cyst – 5148582   160(26)
Eyelid, lower, drooping – 5142321   161(08)
Eyelid, upper, drooping – 18543121   163(26)

F

Fainting spells – 4854548   126(11)
Famine dropsy – 5456784   70(29)
Farsightedness – 5189988   161(34)
Farsightedness of the aging – 1481854   163(18)
Fascioliasis – 4812542   90(09)
Favism – 54321457   76(26)
Favus – 4851481   135(26)
Fetal alcohol syndrome – 4845421   103(07)
Fever, spotted – 5189499   96(15)
Fibroadenoma, breast – 4854312   143(19)
Fibrocystic breasts – 4851432   142(13)
Fibroids, uterine – 51843216   117(31)

Fibroma, nasopharynx – 1111122	154(25)
Fibrosis, progressive – 1110006	55(01)
Fig warts – 1489543	134(30)
Fistula, anal – 5189421	143(28)
Fistula, epithelial coccygeal – 9018532	143(22)
Fistula, rectal – 5189421	143(28)
Fistula, tracheoesophageal – 514854714	151(12)
Fixed ideas – 8142543	130(19)
Flat feet – 1891432	143(34)
Flu – 4814212	91(24)
Food allergy – 2841482	65(05)
Food poisoning – 5184231	90(13)
Foot and mouth disease – 9912399	90(18)
Foreign object aspiration – 4821543	103(12)
Foreign objects	
bronchi – 5485432	144(03)
ear – 54321545	155(15)
esophagus – 14854321	144(07)
soft tissue – 148543297	144(11)
stomach – 8184321	144(15)
Fracture – 7776551	144(19)
Frigidity, female – 5148222	132(19)
Frostbite – 4858514	144(22)
Funicular myelitis – 518543251	122(05)
Furuncle – 5148385	144(25)
Furuncle, nasal vestibule – 1389145	155(20)

G

Galactosemia – 48125421	103(16)
Gas gangrene – 41543218	144(28)
Gastric atony, acute – 5485671	66(03)
Gastritis	
acute – 4567891	65(13)
chronic – 5489120	65(19)

gastritis – 5485674 — 65(09)
Gastrocardial syndrome – 5458914 — 65(23)
Gastrointestinal tuberculosis – 8143215 — 65(34)
Gastroparesis – 5485671 — 66(03)
Gastroptosis – 81234574 — 63(01)
Gaucher's disease – 5145432 — 76(31)
Gender differentiation, congenital disorders of – 5451432 — 81(07)
Genital warts – 1489543 — 134(30)
German measles – 4218547 — 94(14)
Giant-cell Arteritis – 9998102 — 53(16)
Giardiasis – 5189148 — 90(23)
Gingivitis – 548432123 — 166(04)
Glaucoma – 5131482 — 161(25)
Glomerulonephritis
    acute – 4285614 — 72(23)
    diffuse proliferative GN – 4812351 — 72(19)
    glomerulonephritis – 8491454 — 53(22)
    in children – 5145488 — 103(20)
Glossalgia – 514852181 — 166(07)
Glossitis – 1484542 — 166(10)
Glottis, edema of – 2314514 — 155(24)
Goiter, endemic – 5432178 — 81(11)
Goiter, exophthalmic – 5143218 — 81(15)
Goiter, toxic diffuse (Graves' disease) – 5143218 — 81(15)
Gonorrhea – 5148314 — 117(01)
Gonorrhea, in men – 2225488 — 135(30)
Goodpasture's syndrome – 8491454 — 53(22)
Gout – 8543215 — 54(09)
Grandiosity – 148454283 — 129(06)
Granulomatosis, Wegener's – 8943568 — 55(29)
Growth hormone deficiency – 4141414 — 81(19)
Guillain-Barré syndrome – 4548128 — 125(16)
Gynecomastia – 4831514 — 144(31)

H

Hair loss – 5484121	134(18)
Hallucinosis – 4815428	129(10)
Hallux valgus – 5418521	153(04)
Hamman–Rich syndrome – 4814578	58(07)
Hay fever – 514852351	157(26)
Headache – 4818543	122(10)
Headache, cluster – 4851485	122(13)
Heart attack – 8914325	50(11)
Heart blocks – 9874321	49(16)
Heart defect	
acquired – 8124569	49(19)
congenital – 9995437	48(34)
congenital (childhood) – 14891548	103(23)
Heart disease, rheumatic – 5481543	107(18)
Heart failure – 8542196	49(23)
Heart failure, acute – 1895678	36(17)
Helminthiasis – 5124548	90(28)
Hemangioma – 4812599	109(12)
Hemarthrosis – 4857543	144(33)
Hemarthrosis – 7184321	153(08)
Hematoma, nasal septum – 5431482	155(28)
Hematosarcoma – 54321451	41(23)
Hemoblastosis outside of bone marrow – 54321451	77(01)
Hemochromatosis – 5454589	66(11)
Hemolytic disease of the newborn – 5125432	103(30)
Hemophilia – 548214514	104(01)
Hemorrhage	
during childbirth – 4814821	112(20)
dysfunctional bleeding of the uterus	
– 4853541	117(04)
external – 4321511	145(01)
gastrointestinal – 5121432	110(07)
internal – 5142543	145(06)

Hemorrhagic diathesis
        by pathology of blood vessels – 54815438   77(11)
        hemorrhagic diathesis – 0480421   104(04)
        hemorrhagic diathesis – 5148543   77(08)
Hemorrhagic disease of the newborn – 5128543   104(07)
Hemorrhagic fever with renal syndrome – 5124567   90(32)
Hemorrhagic vasculitis – 8491234   53(28)
Hemorrhoids – 58143219   145(11)
Henoch-Schoenlein purpura – 5128421   106(24)
Hepatic insufficiency – 8143214   66(18)
Hepatic steatosis – 5143214   67(20)
Hepatitis
        acute – 58432141   66(24)
        chronic – 5123891   66(31)
        hepatitis – 5814243   66(22)
        viral, A und B – 5412514   91(01)
Hepatocerebral dystrophy – 48143212   122(17)
Hepatolenticular degeneration – 48143212   122(17)
Hepatolenticular degeneration – 5438912   67(01)
Hepatolienalic syndrome – 8451485   67(27)
Hepatopathy, toxic – 48145428   86(19)
Hepatosis
        acute – 1234576   67(11)
        cholestatic – 5421548   67(15)
        chronic – 5143214   67(20)
Hepatosis – 9876512   67(06)
Hepatosplenomegalic lipoidosis – 4851888   67(24)
Hepatosplenomegaly syndrome – 8451485   67(27)
Hernia
        congenital diaphragmatic – 518543257   151(17)
        diaphragmatic – 5189412   110(11)
        hernia – 95184321   145(14)
Herniated disk – 5481321   125(25)
Herpes simplex – 2312489   91(08)
Herpes zoster – 51454322   122(24)

Herpes, oral and genital – 2312489	91(08)
Hiatal spasm – 4895132	60(07)
Hidradenitis – 4851348	145(17)
High blood pressure – 8145432	49(27)
Histiocytosis, x-type – 5484321	104(13)
HIV – 5148555	91(13)
Hives – 1858432	139(12)
Hodgkin's lymphoma – 4845714	77(31)
Hookworm infestation – 4815454	87(20)
Hordeolum – 514854249	161(31)
Horton's disease – 9998102	53(16)
Human immunodeficiency virus – 5148555	91(13)
Hunger edema – 5456784	70(29)
Hydramnios – 5123481	113(33)
Hydrocele, spermatic cord – 481543255	145(22)
Hydrocele, testis – 481543255	145(22)
Hydrocephalus – 81432143	122(28)
Hydronephrosis – 5432154	72(25)
Hydrophobia – 4812543	91(19)
Hymenolepiasis – 54812548	91(21)
Hyperacidity, stomach – 5484214	63(24)
Hyperbilirubinemia	
benign – 84514851	67(31)
congenital – 8432180	68(03)
posthepatic – 8214321	68(07)
Hyperesthesia, teeth – 1484312	166(13)
Hyperinsulinemia – 48454322	81(23)
Hyperlipidemia, idiopathic – 4851888	68(12)
Hyperliproteinemia – 4851888	67(24)
Hyperopia – 5189988	161(34)
Hyperparathyroidism – 5481412	82(17)
Hyperprolactinemia – 4812454	81(29)
Hypersexuality – 5414855	132(22)
Hypertension – 8145432	49(27)
Hypertension, portal – 8143218	70(04)

Hypertensive crisis – 5679102   49(30)
Hypervitaminosis D – 5148547   104(17)
Hypochondria – 1488588   129(15)
Hypogalactia – 48123147   112(29)
Hypogonadism (male) – 48143121   81(33)
Hypoparathyroidism – 4514321   82(01)
Hypophyseal dwarfism – 4141414   81(19)
Hypopituitarism – 48143214   82(06)
Hypoplasia, tooth enamel – 74854321   166(16)
Hypoprothrombinemia – 5481542   77(16)
Hypotension – 8143546   50(01)
Hypothalamic syndrome – 514854215   121(25)
Hypothyroidism – 4512333   104(21)
Hypothyroidism – 4812415   82(11)
Hypovitaminosis – 5154231   98(15)
Hysterical syndrome – 5154891   129(19)

I

Ichthyosis – 9996789   136(01)
Icterus – 5432148   68(34)
Icterus neonatorum – 4815457   104(33)
Ileocecal valve inflammation – 58432148   68(22)
Ileus, paralytic – 4548148   145(24)
Impotence – 8851464   132(25)
Impotence, erectile dysfunction – 184854281   132(14)
Indigestion – 1112223   63(19)
Indigestion – 9988771   68(25)
Infantile tetany – 5148999   104(24)
Infarction, pulmonary – 89143211   58(21)
Infectious arthritis – 8111110   53(33)
Infertility – 9918755   117(09)
Inflammation, large intestine – 8454321   61(30)
Influenza, seasonal – 4814212   91(24)
Ingested poisons – 5142154   85(13)

Ingrown nail – 4548547 — 145(28)
Inhaled poisons – 4548142 — 85(17)
Injected poisons– 4818142 — 85(20)
Insufficiency of the cardiac sphincter – 8545142 — 68(29)
Intestinal stasis – 4548148 — 145(24)
Intracranial birth trauma – 518999981 — 104(29)
Intussusception – 5148231 — 110(17)
Invagination – 5148231 — 110(17)
Iritis – 5891231 — 162(04)
Iron deficiency anemia – 1458421 — 100(28)
Iron overload disease – 5454589 — 66(11)
Ischemic heart disease (IHD) – 1454210 — 50(05)
Ischuria, acute – 0144444 — 150(03)
Itching – 1249812 — 137(16)
Itsenko Cushing syndrome – 54321458 — 80(21)

J

Jaundice
    jaundice – 5432148 — 68(34)
    neonatal – 4815457 — 104(33)
    obstructive – 8012001 — 145(32)
    obstructive – 8214321 — 68(07)
Jaw, fractured – 5182148 — 166(19)
Joint disease, degenerative – 8145812 — 52(17)

K

Keratitis – 518432114 — 162(07)
Kidney
Kidney colic – 4321054 — 73(14)
Kidney disease, chronic – 5488821 — 72(30)
Kidney failure – 4321843 — 73(22)
Kidney failure, acute – 8218882 — 73(28)
Kidney failure, chronic – 5488821 — 72(30)

Kidney stones – 5432143   72(33)
Kidney damage – 5412123   86(14)
Kissing disease – 5142548   92(34)
Korsakoff's syndrome – 4185432   129(23)
Kraurosis vulvae – 58143218   117(13)
Kussmaul disease – 54321894   54(13)

L

Labor, abnormal patterns during – 14891543   112(24)
Labyrinthitis – 48154219   155(31)
Lactose intolerance – 4845432   64(03)
Lambliasis – 5189148   90(23)
Laryngeal membrane – 148543283   156(01)
Laryngeal web – 148543283   156(01)
Laryngitis
         allergic – 58143214   105(01)
         laryngitis – 4548511   156(05)
         subglottic – 1489542   106(19)
Laryngomalacia – 4185444   158(14)
Laryngospasm – 485148248   156(07)
Laryngotracheobronchitis – 1489542   106(19)
Lazy eye – 1899999   160(10)
Legionellosis – 5142122   91(27)
Legionnaires' disease – 5142122   91(27)
Leiomyoma – 55114214   146(01)
Leishmaniasis – 5184321   91(33)
Lens displacement – 25184321   161(04)
Leprosy – 148543294   136(04)
Leptospirosis – 5128432   92(04)
Leukemia – 5481347   77(20), 105(06)
Leukemia, chronic myeloid – 5142357   78(01)
Leukemoid reactions – 5814321   77(24)
Leukoderma – 4812588   136(06)

Leukoplakia – 485148151	166(22)
Leukoplakia, vulva or cervix – 5185321	117(17)
Leukorrhea (Vaginal discharge) – 5128999	117(23)
Lice, infestation of – 48148121	93(28)
Lichen ruber planus – 4858415	136(11)
Lipodystrophy, intestinal – 4814548	69(10)
Lipoma – 4814842	146(04)
Listeriosis – 5812438	92(08)
Liver cirrhosis – 4812345	61(22)
Liver damage – 48145428	86(19)
Liver damage, toxic – 1234576	67(11)
Liver failure – 8143214	66(18)
Liver fluke, Chinese – 5412348	88(25)
Liver, fatty – 5143214	67(20)
Lockjaw, tetanus – 5671454	95(17)
Lou Gehrig's disease – 5148910	120(17)
Low blood pressure – 8143546	50(01)
Lues – 1484999	50(01)
Lung	
cancer – 4541589	58(12)
candidiasis – 4891444	58(16)
edema – 54321112	51(01)
fibrosis – 9871234	57(13)
infarction – 89143211	58(21)
Lupus erythematosus – 8543148	54(01)
Luxation – 5123145	146(07)
Lyell's syndrome – 4891521	136(15)
Lymphadenitis – 4542143	146(09)
Lymphadenitis, subacute regional – 48145421	88(18)
Lymphangitis – 484851482	146(12)
Lymphatic predisposition – 5148548	105(08)
Lymphogranulomatosis – 4845714	41(30)
Lymphogranulomatosis inguinalis – 1482348	136(20)
Lymphoma (Lymphocytoma) – 54321451	41(23)
Lymphoma of the skin – 5891243	41(34)

Lyssa – 4812543   92(12)

M

Malabsorption – 48543215	69(20)
Malabsorption syndrome – 4518999	105(13)
Malaria – 5189999	92(14)
Malta fever – 4122222	88(10)
Manic-depressive disorder – 514218857	128(24)
Marburg hemorrhagic fever – 5184599	92(18)
Marburg virus disease – 5184599	92(18)
Marchiafava-Micheli syndrome – 5481455	78(20)
Marie-Struempell disease – 4891201	55(06)
Mastitis – 8152142	146(15)
Mastitis, newborns – 514854238	151(29)
Mastocytosis – 148542171	136(23)
Mastoiditis, acute – 514832186	156(11)
Mastoiditis, chronic – 1844578	156(32)
Mastopathy – 84854321	146(18)
Measles – 4214825	94(19)
Meckel's diverticulum – 4815475	110(21)
Mediastinitis – 4985432	146(21)
Megacolon – 4851543	146(25)
Megaesophagus – 4895132	60(07)
Melanoma – 5674321	42(03)
Meniere's disease – 514854233	156(15)
Meningitis – 51485431	122(33)
Meningococcal infection – 5891423	92(24)
Meniscus tear – 8435482	146(29)
Menopause – 4851548	117(27)
Mental confusion – 4518533	129(27)
Mental retardation – 1857422	130(23)
Mesothelioma – 58912434	42(08)
Metagonimiasis – 54812541	92(29)
Metalloconiosis – 4845584	57(18)

Microsporia – 1858321	137(31)
Microtrauma, repetitive – 4814542	84(23)
Migraine – 4831421	123(01)
Mikulicz disease – 4891456	54(30)
Milk glands, dysfunction of during lactation period – 48123147	112(29)
Mole, hydatidiform – 4121543	112(33)
Mole, vesicular – 4121543	112(33)
Molluscum contagiosum – 514321532	136(26)
Mononeuropathy – 4541421	123(04)
Mononucleosis, infectious – 5142548	92(34)
Motor neuron disease – 5148910	120(17)
Mucocele, frontal sinus – 5148322	156(19)
Mucoviscidosis – 9154321	101(22)
Multiple Sclerosis – 51843218	123(07)
Mumps – 3218421	93(23)
Muscular dystrophy, progressive – 85432183	123(12)
Musculoskeletal system, diseases in newborns – 514218873	151(32)
Myasthenia gravis – 9987542	123(16)
Mycoplasma – 5481111	93(05)
Mycosis fungoides – 4814588	136(29)
Mydriasis – 18543211	120(13)
Myelitis – 4891543	123(20)
Myelocytosis – 5142357	78(01)
Myelopathia – 51843219	123(24)
Myocardial infarction – 8914325	50(11)
Myocardiodystrophy – 8432110	50(17)
Myocardiopathy – 8421432	48(11)
Myocarditis – 85432104	50(21)
Myoma, uterine – 51843216	117(31)
Myopia – 548132198	162(09)
Myotonia congenita – 4848514	123(28)
Myotonic dystrophy – 481543244	123(33)
Myxedema – 4812415	82(11)

N

Nail infection – 8999999   147(12)
Nail, ingrown – 4548547   145(28)
Narcolepsy – 48543216   124(05)
Narcomania – 5333353   129(32)
Narcomania and Toxicomania – 1414551   130(06)
Narcotics, addiction to – 5333353   129(32)
Nearsightedness – 548132198   162(09)
Negative (deficit) symptoms – 5418538   130(10)
Neonatal sepsis – 4514821   107(32)
Nephritis, hereditary – 5854312   105(18)
Nephrolithiasis – 5432143   72(33)
Nephropathy, salt-losing – 3245678   107(07)
Nephropathy, toxic – 5412123   86(14)
Nerve root syndrome – 5481321   125(25)
Neuralgia – 4541421   123(04)
Neuritis – 4541421   123(04)
Neuritis, optic – 5451589   162(13)
Neuroblastoma – 8914567   42(11)
Neurocirculatory dystonia – 5432150   50(24)
Neurodermatitis – 1484857   136(32)
Neurodermitis, diffuse – 5484215   135(05)
Neuroma, acoustic – 518999955   124(10)
Neuropathy, facial nerves – 518999955   124(10)
Neurorheumatism – 8185432   124(14)
Neurosyphilis – 5482148   124(17)
Neurotic disorder – 48154211   130(15)
Neutropenia – 4856742   75(10)
Neutropenia, congenital – 8432145   78(04)
Niacin deficiency – 1842157   99(06)
Night blindness – 5142842   162(18)
Nose bleeds – 65184321   155(08)
Nyctalopia – 5142842   162(18)

O

Obesity – 4812412	82(14)
Obsessive compulsive disorder – 8142543	130(19)
Obstructive jaundice – 8214321	68(07)

Occlusion

central retinal artery – 514852178	162(21)
central retinal vein – 7777788	162(25)
of major arteries – 81543213	146(32)

Occupational diseases

exposure to physical factors – 4514541	84(14)
influence of biological agents – 81432184	84(19)
influence of chemicals – 9916515	84(10)
overexertion of individual organs, systems – 4814542	84(23)

Ocular burn – 8881112	162(30)
Ocular hypertension – 5131482	161(25)
Oligophrenia – 1857422	130(23)
Omphalocele – 5143248	110(25)
Onanism (Masturbation) – 0021421	132(28)
Onychocryptosis – 4548547	145(28)
Oophoritis – 5143548	117(34)
Ophthalmia, sympathetic – 8185321	162(34)
Ophthalmoplegia – 4848532	124(21)
Opisthorchiasis – 5124542	93(11)
Optic disc edema – 145432152	163(11)
Optic nerve, atrophy – 5182432	163(03)
Orchiepididymitis – 818432151	147(01)
Ornithosis (Psittacosis) – 5812435	93(15)
Osteoarthritis – 8145812	52(17)
Osteoarthrosis – 8145812	52(17)
Osteodystrophia fibrosa – 5481412	82(17)

Osteomyelitis

acute hematogenous in newborns – 5141542	152(01)

epiphyseal – 12345895	110(30)
jawbone – 5414214	166(26)
traumatic – 514854221	147(04)
Othematoma– 4853121	156(23)
Otitis (externa, media, interna) – 55184321	156(28)
Otoantritis – 1844578	156(32)
Otomycosis – 514832188	157(01)
Otosclerosis – 4814851	157(04)
Otospongiosis – 4814851	157(04)
Ovalocytosis, hereditary – 51454323	78(09)
Ovarian apoplexy – 1238543	118(03)
Overexertion, chronic – 4814542	84(23)
Ozaena – 514854241	157(08)

P

Pain management during childbirth – 5421555	113(01)
Palatoschisis – 5151515	110(33)
Panaritium – 8999999	147(12)
Pancreas cancer, islet cell – 8951432	43(13)
Pancreatitis, acute – 4881431	147(08)
Pancreatitis, chronic – 5891432	69(27)
Panhypopituitarism – 48143214	82(06)
Panophthalmia – 5141588	163(08)
Papilledema – 145432152	163(11)
Papillitis, interdental – 5844522	166(30)
Paradontosis – 58145421	167(01)
Paralysis	
familial periodic – 5123488	124(25)
laryngeal – 1854555	157(13)
progressive – 512143223	130(27)
Parametritis – 5143215	118(08)
Parapertussis – 2222221	93(19)
Paraproctitis, acute – 4842118	152(04)
Parathyroid tetany – 4514321	82(01)

Paratyphoid fever – 1411111   96(04)
Parkinson's disease – 54811421   124(29)
Parkinsonism – 54811421   124(29)
Paronychia – 8999999   147(12)
Parotitis epidemica – 3218421   93(23)
Paroxysmal nocturnal hemoglobinuria (PNH)
    – 5481455   78(20)
Pediculosis – 48148121   93(28)
Pelvis
    narrow – 2148543   113(07)
    narrow (anatomically) – 4812312   113(11)
    narrow (clinically) – 4858543   113(15)
Pemphigus – 8145321   137(01)
Peptic ulcer disease of the stomach and duodenum
    – 8125432   69(31)
Percutaneous poisoning – 4814823   85(10)
Periarteritis nodosa – 54321894   54(13)
Periarthritis – 4548145   54(05)
Pericarditis – 9996127   50(34)
Pericoronitis – 5188888   166(33)
Periodontal disease – 58145421   167(01)
Periodontitis – 5182821   167(07)
Periodontitis, apical – 3124601   167(12)
Peritonitis – 1428543   147(15)
Peritonitis, newborns – 4184321   152(08)
Pertussis – 4812548   93(32)
Pes planus – 1891432   143(34)
Pfeiffer's disease – 5142548   92(34)
Phakomatoses – 5142314   125(01)
Pharyngeal fistula – 514854214   142(08)
Pharyngitis – 1858561   157(17)
Pharyngomycosis – 1454511   157(20)
Phenylketonuria – 5148321   105(23)
Pheochromocytoma – 4818145   82(21)
Phimosis, Paraphimosis – 0180010   147(20)

Phlebothrombosis – 1454580   147(25)
Phlegmon
         maxillofacial region – 5148312   167(17)
         necrotic cutaneous, in newborns – 514852173   152(14)
         newborns – 51485433   111(01)
         phlegmon – 48143128   147(29)
         stomach – 4567891   71(01)
Photo ophthalmia – 5841321   163(14)
Photokeratitis – 5841321   163(14)
Pigment cirrhosis – 5454589   61(27)
Pityriasis rosea – 5148315   137(06)
Pityriasis versicolor – 18543214   137(09)
Placenta praevia – 1481855   113(21)
Placental abruption – 1111155   113(25)
Plague – 8998888   94(01)
Platypodia – 1891432   143(34)
Pleurisy – 4854444   57(24)
Pleuritis – 4854444   57(24)
Pleuritis, purulent – 514854223   143(10)
Pneumatosis, gastric – 54321455   70(01)
Pneumoconiosis – 8423457   57(28)
Pneumoconiosis of organic dust – 4548912   57(33)
Pneumonia
         atypical – 5481111   93(05)
         chronic – 51421543   105(27)
         neonatal – 5151421   106(01)
         pneumonia – 4814489   58(01)
         walking – 5481111   93(05)
Pneumonitis, acute interstitial – 4814578   58(07)
Pneumonitis, hypersensitive – 51843215   106(04)
Pneumosclerosis – 9871234   57(13)
Pneumothorax – 5142147   151(23)
Pneumothorax, spontaneous – 481854221   147(32)
Podagra – 8543215   54(09)
Poisonings, acute

ingestion – 5142154	85(13)
inhalation – 4548142	85(17)
injected – 4818142	85(20)
percutaneous – 4814823	85(10)
scorpion stings – 4188888	85(28)
snakebite – 4114111	85(32)
snakebites, other poisonous arthropods – 4812521	85(24)
tarantula spider bites – 8181818	86(01)
wasp and bee stings – 9189189	86(06)
Poliomyelitis (Paralysis, infantile) – 2223214	125(05)
Pollinosis – 514852351	157(26)
Polyarteritis nodosa – 54321894	54(13)
Polyavitaminosis – 4815432	98(20)
Polycystic kidney disease (PKD) – 5421451	73(01)
Polycystic Ovarian Disease – 518543248	118(11)
Polyhydramnios – 5123481	113(33)
Polymyositis – 5481234	53(12)
Polyneuropathy – 4838514	125(11)
Polyneuropathy, acute inflammatory demyelinating – 4548128	125(16)
Polyp	
cervical or uterine – 518999973	118(16)
nasal – 5519740	157(23)
polyp – 4819491	148(01)
Portal Hypertension – 45143211	106(11)
Portal hypertension – 8143218	70(04)
Postcholecystectomy syndrome – 4518421	148(05)
Post-hepatitis syndrome – 4812819	70(08)
Post-lumbar puncture syndrome – 818543231	125(21)
Postnatal period, normal – 12891451	114(01)
Postpartum complications – 41854218	114(04)
Postpartum period – 12891451	114(01)
Potter's rot – 4818912	58(34)
Predisposition to allergies – 0195451	100(14)

Pre-eclampsia – 1848542   115(04)
Pregnancy
        birth and due date – 1888711   114(09)
        ectopic (restoration of health, retention of
        the fetus) – 4812311   114(16)
        multiple – 123457854   114(21)
        post-term (prolonged) – 5142148   114(24)
        uterine – 1899911   114(27)
Premenstrual syndrome (PMS) – 9917891   118(20)
Presbyopia – 1481854   163(18)
Preterm birth – 1284321   114(31)
Prolapse, uterus and vagina – 514832183   118(25)
Proptosis – 5454311   161(18)
Prostatitis – 9718961   148(09)
Prostrate adenoma – 51432144   148(12)
Prurigo nodularis – 5189123   137(12)
Pruritus – 1249812   137(16)
Pruritus vulvae – 5414845   118(30)
Pseudarthrosis – 4814214   148(16)
Pseudarthrosis – 8214231   153(10)
Pseudocroup – 1489542   106(19)
Pseudocroup – 5148523   106(17)
Pseudohypoaldosteronism – 3245678   107(07)
Psoriasis – 999899181   137(21)
Psychiatric disease from toxic exposure – 9977881   86(25)
Psychic defect – 8885512   130(31)
Psychoneurotic disorder from toxic exposure – 9977881   86(25)
Psychoorganic syndrome – 51843212   131(01)
Psychopathic disorder – 4182546   131(04)
Psychoses, symptomatic – 8148581   131(09)
Psychosexual disorder – 0001112   132(31)
Psychosis
        involutional – 18543219   131(14)
        presenile – 18543219   131(14)
        reactive – 0101255   131(20)

senile – 481854383   131(24)
Psychotic disorder, substance-induced – 1142351   131(28)
Pterygium – 18543212   163(23)
Ptosis – 18543121   163(26)
Puberal juvenile dyspituitarism syndrome – 4145412   81(01)
Puberty, premature – 4814312   82(26)
Pulmonary cancer – 4541589   58(12)
Pulmonary candidiasis – 4891444   58(16)
Pulmonary edema – 54321112   51(01)
Pulmonary gangrene – 4838543   148(21)
Pulmonary heart disease – 5432111   49(05)
Pulmonary hemorrhage – 8491454   53(22)
Pulmonary infarction – 89143211   58(21)
Pulmonary tuberculosis – 8941234   59(07)
Pulpitis – 1468550   167(21)
Pupillotonia – 18543211   120(13)
Purpura Henoch-Schoenlein – 8491234   53(28)
Purpura rheumatica – 5128421   106(24)
Putnam-Dana syndrome – 518543251   122(05)
Pyelitis – 5432110   73(08)
Pyelonephritis – 58143213   73(10)
Pyloric stenosis – 81543211   148(25)
Pyloric stenosis, infant – 5154321   106(30)
Pylorospasm, infant – 5141482   106(34)
Pyoderma – 51432149   137(25)
Pyopneumothorax – 148543299   148(30)
Pyridoxine deficiency – 9785621   99(13)

Q

Q-Fever – 5148542   94(04)

R

Rabies – 4812543   94(08)

Rachitis – 5481232   107(27)
Radiation sickness, acute – 481543294   78(26)
Radiation sickness, chronic – 4812453   78(31)
Radiculitis – 5481321   125(25)
Radiculopathy – 5481321   125(25)
Recklinghausen's Disease – 5481412   82(17)
Rectal prolapse – 514832187   148(33)
Reiter's syndrome – 4848111   52(23)
Renal colic – 4321054   73(14)
Renal diabetes – 5142585   107(03)
Renal Eclampsia – 8149141   73(18)
Renal failure – 4321843   73(22)
Renal failure, acute – 8218882   73(28)
Renal glucosuria – 5142585   107(03)
Renal salt-wasting syndrome – 3245678   107(07)
Renal tuberculosis – 5814543   73(33)
Repetitive strain injury – 4814542   84(23)
Respiratory distress syndrome in newborns – 5148284   107(13)
Respiratory failure, acute – 1257814   36(25)
Respiratory tract infection, upper – 48145488   96(20)
Retinal angiomatosis – 5142314   125(01)
Retinal detachment – 1851760   163(29)
Retinitis – 5484512   163(33)
Retinol deficiency – 4154812   98(23)
Rhabdomyosarcoma in children – 5671254   42(20)
Rhesus disease – 5125432   103(30)
Rheumatic fever – 5481543   51(06)
Rheumatic heart disease – 5481543   51(06)
Rheumatism, soft tissue near joint – 1489123   54(18)
Rheumatoid arthritis – 8914201   52(28)
Rhinitis
         allergic – 514852351   157(26)
         allergic (childhood) – 5814325   107(21)
         atrophic – 514854241   157(08)

rhinitis – 5189912	154(32)
vasomotor – 514852351	157(26)
Rhinoscleroma – 0198514	157(31)
Riboflavin deficiency – 1485421	99(01)
Rickets – 5481232	107(27)
Ringing in the ear – 1488513	158(17)
Ringworm	
Epidermophyton – 5148532	137(28)
from dogs and cats (Microsporum) – 1858321	137(31)
Trichophytosis – 4851482	138(01)
Roemheld syndrome – 5458914	65(23)
Rosacea – 518914891	138(04)
Rotavirus – 5148567	94(11)
Roundworm infestation – 4814812	87(27)
Rubella – 4218547	94(14)
Rubeola – 4214825	94(19)

S

Salmonellosis – 5142189	94(24)
Salpingitis – 5148914	118(33)
Sarcoidosis – 4589123	58(25)
Sarcoma, Kaposi's – 8214382	42(26)
Sarcoma, soft-tissue – 54321891	42(31)
Scabies – 8132548	138(09)
Scarlatina – 5142485	94(27)
Scarlet fever – 5142485	94(27)
Schistosomiasis – 48125428	94(33)
Schizophrenia – 1858541	131(33)
Schoenlein-Henoch purpura – 5128421	106(24)
Sciatica – 5481321	125(25)
Scleritis – 514854248	164(01)
Scleroma – 0198514	157(31)
Scorpion stings – 4188888	85(28)
Scurvy – 4141255	99(21)
Sebaceous cyst – 888888179	149(01)

Seborrhea – 1234512   138(13)
Sepsis
        acute – 8914321   45(10)
        chronic – 8145421   8145421
        neonatorum – 4514821   45(10)
        otogenic – 5900001   158(01)
Sex differentiation, congenital disorders of – 5451432   81(07)
Sexual development, premature – 4814312   82(26)
Sexual dysfunction
        imaginary – 1484811   133(11)
        neuroendocrine disorders, from
        psychic – 2148222   133(16)
        sexual dysfunction – 1818191   133(01)
Sexual perversion – 0001112   132(31)
Sharp's syndrome – 1484019   52(33)
Shigellosis – 4812148   89(11)
Shingles – 51454322   122(24)
Shock
        exotoxic – 4185421   86(10)
        shock–like conditions – 1895132   37(02)
        traumatic – 1454814   153(14)
        traumatic – 1895132   37(02)
Sicca syndrome – 4891456   54(30)
Siderophilia – 5454589   66(11)
Silicatosis – 2224698   58(31)
Silicosis – 4818912   58(34)
Simmond's disease – 48143214   82(06)
Sinus barotrauma – 514854237   154(17)
Sinusitis – 1800124   158(06)
Sinusitis, allergic (childhood) – 5814325   107(21)
Sjoegren's syndrome – 4891456   54(30)
Skin toxicosis – 514832184   138(17)
Skin, poisoning through – 4814823   85(10)
Skleroderma, systemic – 1110006   55(01)
Sleep disorder – 514248538   125(30)
Smallpox – 4848148   96(30)

Snakebite – 4114111	85(32)
Snow blindness – 5841321	163(14)
Soft chancre – 4815451	139(08)
Somatosensory amplification – 1488588	129(15)
Spasmophilia – 5148999	104(24)
Spasms – 51245424	104(24)
Spinal amyotrophy – 5483312	125(34)
Spinal apoplexy – 8888881	126(04)
Spinal insult – 8888881	126(04)
Spinal stroke syndrome – 4818542	126(07)
Spondylitis ankylopoetica – 4891201	55(06)
Spotted fever – 5189499	96(15)
Sprains – 5148517	153(18)
Sprue, nontropical – 4891483	64(12)
Sprue, tropical – 5481215	70(23)
Staphylococcus infection – 5189542	108(01)
Starvation edema – 5456784	70(29)
Steatoma – 888888179	149(01)
Steatorrhea, idiopathic – 4891483	64(12)
Stein-Leventhal syndrome – 518543248	118(11)
Stenocardia – 8145999	51(10)
Stenosis	
duodenal – 5557777	109(19)
laryngeal – 7654321	158(09)
pyloric – 81543211	148(25)
Sterility – 9918755	117(09)
Steven-Johnson syndrome – 9814753	138(22)
Stomach ulcers, symptomatic – 9671428	71(04)
Stomatitis – 4814854	167(25)
Stomatocytosis, hereditary – 4814581	79(01)
Strabismus – 518543254	164(06)
Stridor, congenital – 4185444	158(14)
Stroke – 4818542	126(07)
Strongyloidiasis – 54812527	95(04)
Strumitis – 4811111	82(30)

Stye – 514854249   161(31)
Subfebrile condition in children – 5128514   108(05)
Subperiostal hemorrhage – 48543214   109(34)
Subsepsis allergica – 5421238   108(10)
Sucrose intolerance – 4845432   64(03)
Superior mesenteric artery (SMA) syndrome – 5891234   71(08)
Surfer's eye – 18543212   163(23)
Syncope – 4854548   126(11)
Synechia, nasal – 1989142   154(28)
Syphilis – 1484999   138(27)
Syringomyelia – 1777771   126(16)
Systemic vasculitis (SV) – 1894238   55(11)

T

Taeniarhynchosis – 4514444   95(09)
Taeniasis – 4855555   95(12)
Takayasu's arteritis – 8945432   55(16)
Talcosis – 4845145   59(04)
Talipes equinovarus – 485143241   149(04)
Tapeworm infestation
        beef tapeworm – 4514444   95(09)
        broad tapeworm – 4812354   89(07)
        dwarf tapeworm – 54812548   91(21)
        Echinococcosis – 5481235   89(20)
        fish tapeworm – 4812354   89(07)
        pork tapeworm – 4855555   95(12)
        small fox tapeworm – 5481454   87(10)
Tarantula spider bite – 8181818   86(01)
Tears in external genitals during childbirth – 148543291   114(34)
Temporal arteritis – 9998102   53(16)
Tendinitis (see Rheumatism, soft tissue) – 1489123   54(33)
Tendovaginitis – 1489154   55(21)
Tendovaginitis (see Rheumatism, soft tissue) – 1489123 54(33)
Teratoma, sacrococcygeal region – 481543238   111(10)

Tetanus – 5671454	95(17)
Tetany, hypocalcemic – 5148999	104(24)
Tetany, infantile – 5148999	104(24)
Thalassemia – 7765437	79(05)
Thiamine deficiency – 1234578	98(28)
Thomsen's disease – 4848514	123(28)
Thrombangiitis obliterans – 5432142	149(08)
Thrombangiitis obliterans – 8945482	55(24)
Thromboarteriitis – 8945482	55(24)
Thrombocytopathy – 5418541	79(10)
Thrombophilia, hematogenous – 4814543	79(14)
Thrombophlebitis – 1454580	149(14)
Thrombophlebitis – 8945482	55(24)
Thrush – 54842148	61(03)
Thrush – 9876591	134(25)
Thyroiditis – 4811111	82(30)
Tick-borne typhus – 5189499	96(15)
Tinnitus – 1488513	158(17)
TMJ (temporomandibular joint), dislocation– 5484311	168(01)
TMJ (temporomandibular joint), locked jaw – 5484311	168(01)
TMJ, ankylosis,– 514852179	167(28)
TMJ, arthritis – 548432174	167(33)
Tongue inflammation – 1484542	166(10)
Tongue pain – 514852181	166(07)
Tonsil, pharyngeal – 5189514	154(13)
Tonsillar hypertrophy – 4514548	158(20)
Tonsillitis, acute – 1999999	158(24)
Tonsillitis, chronic – 35184321	158(27)
Tonsils, enlarged – 4514548	158(20)
Tooth decay – 5148584	165(30)
Tooth luxation – 485143277	168(05)
Tooth, fractured (broken) – 814454251	168(09)
Toothache, acute – 5182544	168(12)
Torticollis – 4548512	149(16)
Toxemia, in pregnancy – 1848542	115(04)

Toxic hemolytic anemia – 45481424   100(33)
Toxic syndrome – 5148256   108(14)
Toxicosis with exsiccosis – 5148256   108(14)
Toxicosis, psychoneurotic – 9977881   86(25)
Toxoplasmosis – 8914755   95(22)
Tracheitis, allergic – 514854218   108(19)
Trachoma – 5189523   164(10)
Trauma, ear – 4548515   158(30)
Trauma, inner organs – 5432188   153(22)
Trauma, inner organs – 8914319   149(20)
Traumatic shock – 1895132   37(02)
Tremor – 3148567   126(21)
Trichinellosis – 7777778   95(26)
Trichocephalosis – 4125432   95(29)
Trichophyton rubrum – 4518481   138(31)
Trichostrongylosis – 9998888   95(33)
Trichuriasis – 4125432   95(29)
Trigeminal neuralgia – 5148485   126(25)
Troisier-Hanot-Chauffard syndrome – 5454589   66(11)
Tropia – 518543254   164(06)
Tuberculosis
         asymptomatic – 1284345   108(27)
         bone – 148543281   149(23)
         cutaneous – 148543296   139(01)
         gastrointestinal – 8143215   65(34)
         genital – 8431485   119(01)
         in children – 5148214   108(23)
         kidney – 5814543   73(33)
         laryngeal – 5148541   158(33)
         latent – 1284345   108(27)
         pulmonary – 8941234   59(07)
         renal – 5814543   73(33)
Tularemia – 4819489   96(01)
Tumor
         adrenal – 5678123   43(01)

brain – 5451214	126(29)
brain or spinal cord – 5431547	43(09)
islet cell – 8951432	43(13)
larynx – 5148742	159(01)
multiple myeloma – 8432184	42(16)
nasal cavity and paranasal sinuses – 8514256	43(18)
nasopharynx – 5678910	43(22)
non-Hodgkin lymphoma – 8432184	42(16)
paraproteinemia producing tumors – 8432184	78(14)
parathyroid – 1548910	43(26)
peripheral nervous system – 514832182	43(31)
plasmocytoma – 8432184	42(16)
skin – 1458914	139(05)
spinal cord – 51843210	44(01)
tumors, endocrine system – 4541548	82(34)
uterus – 9817453	44(04)
Typhoid fever – 1411111	96(04)
Typhus, epidemic – 1444444	96(10)
Typhus, Queensland tick typhus – 5189499	96(15)

U

Ulcer

corneal – 548432194	164(13)
duodenum, penetrating – 8143291	149(30)
duodenum, penetrating – 9148532	149(26)
peptic, stomach and duodenum – 8125432	69(31)
small intestine, simple nonspecific – 48481452	71(13)
stomach, penetrating – 8143291	149(30)
stomach, penetrating – 9148532	149(26)
stomach, symptomatic – 9671428	71(04)
trophic – 514852154	149(34)
Ulcus molle – 4815451	139(08)
Umbilical cord wound care for newborns – 0123455	115(11)

Umbilical cord, prolapse – 1485432   115(17)
Upper respiratory tract infection – 48145488   96(20)
Uremia, chronic – 8914381   74(04)
Urethritis – 1387549   74(07)
Urinary retention, acute – 0144444   150(03)
Urinary system, anomalies – 1234571   74(10)
Urolithiasis – 5432143   72(33)
Urticaria – 1858432   139(12)
Uveitis – 548432198   164(18)

V

Vaginismus – 5142388   133(20)
Vaginitis – 5148533   119(06)
Varicella – 48154215   96(25)
Varicocele – 81432151   150(08)
Varicosis – 4831388   150(12)
Variola – 4848148   96(30)
Variola minor – 4848148   97(01)
Vascular crisis – 8543218   51(24)
Vascular insufficiency – 8668888   51(30)
Vasculitides, cutaneous – 5142544   139(16)
Vasculitis – 1454231   139(20)
Vasculitis, allergic or hemorrhagic – 8491234   53(28)
Vegetovascular dystonia – 8432910   47(29)
Vernal keratoconjunctivitis (Catarrh, spring)
              – 514258951   164(21)
Verrucae – 5148521   139(24)
Vertigo, cerebral – 514854217   127(09)
Vibration disease – 4514541   84(14)
Virilism – 89143212   83(04)
Vitamin A deficiency – 4154812   98(23)
Vitamin B1 deficiency – 1234578   98(28)
Vitamin B2 deficiency – 1485421   99(01)
Vitamin B3 deficiency – 1842157   99(06)

Vitamin B6 deficiency – 9785621	99(13)
Vitamin C deficiency – 4141255	99(21)
Vitamin D deficiency – 5421432	99(24)
Vitamin D deficiency, rickets – 5481232	107(27)
Vitamin deficiency syndrome – 5451234	98(10)
Vitamin K deficiency – 4845414	99(28)
Vitamin PP deficiency – 1842157	99(06)
Vitiligo – 4812588	136(06)
Vomiting – 1454215	108(32)
Vulva, itchy – 5414845	118(30)
Vulvitis – 5185432	119(09)
Vulvovaginitis – 5814513	119(12)

W

Warts – 5148521	139(24)
Wasp stings – 9189189	86(06)
Wegener's Granulomatosis – 8943568	55(29)
Weil's disease – 5128432	92(04)
Whipple's disease – 4814548	71(19)
Whooping cough – 4812548	93(32)
Wilson's disease – 48143212	122(17)
Wilson-Konowalow disease – 5438912	67(01)
Wissler's syndrome – 5421238	108(10)
Wounds – 5148912	150(16)
Wounds, bleeding – 4321511	145(01)
Wrestler's ear – 4853121	156(23)
Wryneck – 4548512	149(16)

X

Xerostomia – 5814514	168(17)

Y

Yeast infection – 54842148   61(03)
Yeast infection – 9876591   134(25)
Yersinia pseudotuberculosis – 514854212   97(04)
Yersiniosis – 5123851   97(09)

Z

Zollinger-Ellison syndrome – 148543295   150(19)

Diagnosis	Restorative Sequence

Diagnosis	Restorative Sequence

Diagnosis	Restorative Sequence

Diagnosis	Restorative Sequence

Diagnosis	Restorative Sequence